Supportive and Palliative Care and Quality of Life in Oncology

Edited by Bassam Abdul Rasool Hassan

Published in London, United Kingdom

Supportive and Palliative Care and Quality of Life in Oncology
http://dx.doi.org/10.5772/intechopen.100933
Edited by Bassam Abdul Rasool Hassand

Assistant to the Editor: Ali Haider Mohammed

Contributors
Delgersuren Gelegjamts, Batbagana Burenerdene, Neeraj Gour, Meenakshi Chaudhary, Metin Dincer, Antonio Carlos Godoy, Katherine Dambrowski, Paula Barrioso, Caroline Anjos, Cristina Martucci, Alessandro Inserra, Aisha Muthanna Shanshal, Sherri Cervantez, Anand Karnad, Matthew Butler, Yuk Chiu Yip, Ka-Huen Yip, Wai-King Tsui, Susana Villa García Ugarte, Luis Enrique Miranda Calderón, Margaret C. Cecil, Michael H. Hart Plumer, Bassam Abdul Rasool Hassan

First published in London, United Kingdom, 2023 by IntechOpen
IntechOpen is the global imprint of INTECHOPEN LIMITED, registered in England and Wales, registration number: 11086078, 5 Princes Gate Court, London, SW7 2QJ, United Kingdom

British Library Cataloguing-in-Publication Data
A catalogue record for this book is available from the British Library

Additional hard and PDF copies can be obtained from orders@intechopen.com

Supportive and Palliative Care and Quality of Life in Oncology
Edited by Bassam Abdul Rasool Hassan
p. cm.
Print ISBN 978-1-80356-185-1
Online ISBN 978-1-80356-186-8
eBook (PDF) ISBN 978-1-80356-187-5

For EU product safety concerns:
IN TECH d.o.o., Prolaz Marije Krucifikse Kozulić 3, 51000 Rijeka, Croatia,
info@intechopen.com or visit our website at intechopen.com.

Meet the editor

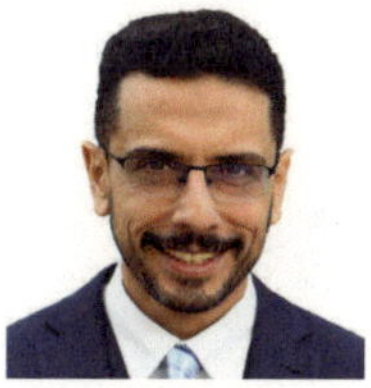

Bassam Abdul Rasool Hassan obtained a Ph.D. in Clinical Pharmacy from the Universiti Sains Malaysia (USM). During 2014–2017, he was a senior lecturer in the Department of Pharmacy, at Universiti Malaya (UM). During 2017–2019, he was a senior lecturer in the Department of Pharmacy Practice, Universiti Teknologi MARA (UiTM), Malaysia. Dr. Hassan is currently a senior lecturer in the Department of Pharmacy, AL-Rafidain University College, Iraq.

Contents

Preface **IX**

Section 1
Quality of Life among Cancer Patients **1**

Chapter 1 **3**
Introductory Chapter: Supportive and Palliative and Quality of Life among Cancer Patients
by Bassam Abdul Rasool Hassan

Chapter 2 **7**
The Quality of Life in Cancer Patients
by Neeraj Gour and Meenakshi Chaudhary

Chapter 3 **17**
Anxiety, Depression, and Delirium in Terminally Ill Cancer Patient
by Susana Villa García Ugarte and Luis Enrique Miranda Calderón

Section 2
Supportive and Palliative Care in Oncology Field **41**

Chapter 4 **43**
Palliative Care for Patients with Lung Cancer: A Review of the Current Developments in the Field and Perspectives on the Implementation of Care
by Yuk-Chiu Yip, Ka-Huen Yip and Wai-King Tsui

Chapter 5 **59**
Supportive and Palliative Care Attitude for Cancer Patients
by Delgersuren Gelegjamts and Batbagana Burenerdene

Chapter 6 **77**
Perspective Chapter: Palliative Surgery in Pediatric Cancer
by Alessandro Inserra and Cristina Martucci

Chapter 7 **93**
Ethics in Palliative Care
by Metin Dincer

Chapter 8 107
Palliative Care Therapies
by Aisha Muthanna Shanshal

Chapter 9 133
Feeding at the End of Life in Brazilian Amazon: Qualitative Analysis of Medical Indications
by Caroline Anjos, Katherine Dambrowski, Antonio Godoy and Paula Barrioso

Chapter 10 145
Leaving Early: The Reality of Assisted Suicide and Euthanasia in 2022
by Michael H. Plumer and Margaret C. Cecil

Chapter 11 175
Prognostic Communication in the Era of Targeted Therapy and Immunotherapy
by Sherri Cervantez, Matthew Butler and Anand Karnad

Preface

The medical terms “supportive and palliative care” and “quality of life” in oncology refer to the two branches of medicine that address the emotional, social, ethical, spiritual, and treatment needs of cancer patients and their families, relatives, and healthcare providers. Additionally, the terms refer to the broader fields of palliative care and medicine that focus on helping individuals (sick and healthy) cope with the unpleasant side effects of cancer and its treatment and the proper way to enhance or maintain quality of life at an acceptable level.

Maintaining or enhancing cancer patients’ quality of life is just as crucial as whatever survival boost a pharmacological or non-pharmacological treatment may offer. Moreover, increased quality of life makes it more likely that patients and their families will stick with their treatments and that recovery will improve.

This book focuses on palliative and supportive care and quality of life to assist physicians, pharmacists, nurses, and researchers in improving their knowledge, awareness, and practice in these areas. It provides up-to-date information and studies focused on these two aspects as they pertain to cancer patients.

Bassam Abdul Rasool Hassan
Department of Pharmacy,
Al-Rafidain University College,
Baghdad, Iraq

Section 1

Quality of Life among Cancer Patients

Chapter 1

Introductory Chapter: Supportive and Palliative and Quality of Life among Cancer Patients

Bassam Abdul Rasool Hassan

1. Introduction

Cancer has risen to prominence as one of the century's leading killers, second only to heart disease in terms of mortality rate. Many scientists are now talking about "lifetime risk" in relation to cancer patients, which might mean either the time it takes for the cancer to develop and spread or the time it takes for the patient to die. Cancer diseases, whether solid or hematological in nature, are accompanied by a plethora of issues (i.e., several side effects).

Therefore, for these reasons, cancer is considered to be one of the most significant diseases that can negatively impact human life expectancy [1].

2. Impact of cancer on patients' quality of life (QoL)

Cancer sufferers' symptoms tend to be quite varied. If symptoms are not properly managed, it can interfere with a person's ability to go about their regular routine. The suffering can be lessened and quality of life (QoL) enhanced through the management of symptoms. Patients with cancer report significant decreases in QoL due to their symptoms. High levels of emotional distress, low levels of physical and social functioning, and a generally lower QoL have all been linked to a greater symptom load. As a result, QoL in cancer patients can be enhanced with careful symptom control [2].

Malathi and colleagues conducted a survey study among 768 Indian patients suffering from several types of solid cancer diseases. The aim was to detect the impact of cancer on patients QoL. Results showed that patients between the ages of 51 and 60 made up 30.2% of the total, and the majority of those patients had head and neck cancer (40.1%), with 57.7% having advanced stages of the disease. Most patients (82.3%) reported that their symptoms reduced their QoL, i.e., cancer disease negatively impacts their QoL [2].

A review study included 82 review articles focused on QoL of breast cancer patients published between 2008 and 2018. The aim was to expand current understanding of how breast cancer affects patients' QoL. Overall, this review showed that the QoL of women with breast cancer has improved over the past decade. The QoL of this cohort was significantly enhanced by a number of relatively straightforward interventions, including increased physical exercise and psychosocial support. However, there are many other aspects that need to be taken into account, including the management of symptoms such as pain and lymphedema, concerns associated to worry, sexual function, especially for young patients, and future outcomes. This review also found that there has been significant progress in addressing methodological concerns related to evaluating QoL in breast cancer patients; however, there is still much work to be done before we have a complete picture of what matters most to these individuals [3].

3. Supportive and palliative care and QoL among cancer patients

A patient's quality of life (QoL) is the primary emphasis of palliative care treatment. The importance of measuring QoL in palliative care is starting to be recognized. QoL is an open-ended concept, with a wide range of interpreted meanings and associated nuances [4].

The physical pain, emotional stress, and financial hardship caused by cancer and its treatment significantly lower the QoL of sufferers (i.e., cancer patients). As a result, in 1990, the WHO launched the palliative care (PC) project, which stands for medical care aimed at enhancing the QoL of people living with life-threatening illnesses by alleviating their symptoms. Assessment, early identification, and treatment of pain, assistance with physical or psychological problems, and spiritual support are all ways in which PC enhances QoL. Patients with cancer often keep taking medications that are no longer helping them because they fear the alternative. Patients with cancer can get the help they need and reduce their symptoms with the right PC approach [5, 6].

Amal and colleagues conducted a prospective study among 240 cancer survivors at King Hussein Cancer Center in Amman, Jordan. The aim was to determine shortage in supportive palliative care and QoL among adult cancer survivors' QoL. Unfortunately, results showed the presence of shortage in several needs of this population, which significantly led to drop down in their QoL [7].

Another prospective study by Antoine and colleagues was conducted in mono-cancer care center in France. The aim was to determine the relationship between meeting their needs (i.e., supportive and palliative care) with both their QoL and decreased unscheduled hospital care. Authors detected that there is a direct relationship between cancer patients QoL and meeting their needs only [8].

Author details

Bassam Abdul Rasool Hassan
Department of Pharmacy, Al-Rafidain University College, Baghdad, Iraq

*Address all correspondence to: bassamsunny@yahoo.com

References

[1] Hassan R. Cancer tragedy in this century and the role of OMICS group open access journal in overcoming this matter. Pharmaceutical Regulatory Affairs. 2012;**1**:1

[2] Nayak MG, George A, Vidyasagar MS, Mathew S, Nayak S, Nayak BS, et al. Quality of life among cancer patients. Indian Journal of Palliative Care. 2017;**23**(4):445-450

[3] Mokhtari-Hessari, Montazeri. Health-related quality of life in breast cancer patients: Review of reviews from 2008 to 2018. Health and Quality of Life Outcomes. 2020;**18**(1):338

[4] Singh DP. Quality of life in cancer patients receiving palliative care. Indian Journal of Palliative Care. 2010;**16**(1):36-43

[5] Gayatri D, Efremov L, Kantelhardt EJ, Mikolajczyk R. Quality of life of cancer patients at palliative care units in developing countries: Systematic review of the published literature. Quality of Life Research. 2021;**30**:315-343

[6] Aboshaiqah A, Al-Saedi TS, Abu-Al-Ruyhaylah MM, Aloufi AA, Alharbi MO, Alharbi SS, et al. Quality of life and satisfaction with care among palliative cancer patients in Saudi Arabia. Palliative & Supportive Care. 2016;**14**(6):621-627

[7] Al-Omari A, Al-Rawashdeh N, Damsees R, Ammar K, Alananzeh I, Inserat B, et al. Supportive care needs assessment for cancer survivors at a Comprehensive Cancer Center in the Middle East: Mending the Gap. Cancers. 2022;**14**(1002):1-19

[8] Arnaud A, Grenier J, Boustany R, Kirscher S, Mege A, de Rauglaudre G, et al. Role of supportive care in improving the quality of life and reducing unscheduled hospital care in patients with metastatic breast cancer. Support Care Cancer. 2021;**29**(7):3735-3742

Chapter 2

The Quality of Life in Cancer Patients

Neeraj Gour and Meenakshi Chaudhary

Abstract

Cancer is a disease mainly caused by uncontrolled division of body cells in any part in the human body. Cancer is epidemiologically one of major non communicable disease and considered to be main health issue in the community across the world. In medicine, we are often interested in how disease or its treatment affects quality of life (QOL), which is generally considered health-related quality of life. All cancer patients should be subjected to attain all dimensions of quality of life i.e. Physical, Mental, Social & Functional Health. QOL is not easy to measure but despite this, there are many models and scales available to assess & ensure QOL among cancer patients. Good QOL also ensures more life expectancy among cancer patients and they can live more social & productive life. Maintenance of good QOL must be integral part of all cancer prevention & treatment.

Keywords: cancer, quality of life (QOL), models of QOL: Scales of QOL, dimensions of QOL

1. Introduction

Cancer is a disease mainly caused by uncontrolled division of body cells in any part in the human body. Normally the cell growth remains under control by the body's immune system. It is the time, when these cells start dividing uncontrollably, forming lumps or growths, that Cancer is caused. Growths like this are called tumors. There are two types of tumors malignant and benign [1].

2. Burden of cancer

Needless to mention that Non-communicable diseases (NCDs) are now well known leading cause of morbidity and mortality worldwide, accounting for approximately 36 million deaths annually around the world, with a rapidly rising prevalence due to population growth and fast changing socio demographic characteristics including aging of population. Moreover, chronically ill patients often suffer from multiple co- morbidities, which can be defined as the co-occurrence of several chronic conditions within one person & one patient [2].

Cancer is epidemiologically one of major non communicable disease and very rapidly becoming to be main health issue in the community around the world. Around the world, cancer is becoming one of the most common causes for morbidity and mortality. Data from GLOBOCAN year 2012 mentions that around 14.1 million new patients were diagnosed with cancer and approximately 8.2 million deaths occurred due to cancer and it is estimated to rise approximately 70% by the year of 2030 [3].

3. What is quality of life (QOL)?

We all have a rolling question all the time that, what is meant by the phrase "quality of life." We know that being free is better than being imprisoned, being healthy is better than being sick, and being relaxed is better than being stressed. There are people who choose to live in the city because they give value access to cultural and social offerings. On the other hand some people choose to live in rural areas because they value the slower pace, lack of traffic, and access to nature. These features affect the inherent goodness of our lives, or our wellbeing, referred to in the medical and scientific arenas as quality of life.

In medicine, we are often interested in how disease or its treatment affects quality of life, which is generally considered health-related quality of life. Health-related quality of life, also abbreviated as HRQOL or HRQL, has evolved over the time into a broad, multidimensional concept that includes both physical and mental health, and also includes social factors.

Quality of life information can be used in different ways in medical practice. Decision of Cancer treatment making is one of the major areas in where quality of life considerations are applied in cancer. For example, a patient and his or her physician may be attempting to decide between two treatments that show virtually no differences in survival or other disease-related outcomes. Quality of life over the time has become deciding factor in selecting one treatment over another. Alternatively, patients may also be provided autonomy to choose two different types of cancer treatment based on the expected toxicity, convenience, or other factors that impact quality of life (**Table 1**).

4. Definition of quality of life

If we talk about root of the QOL concept goes way back to the 1947 World Health Organization (WHO) definition of health as a "state of complete physical, mental and social well-being, and not merely the absence of disease and infirmity [5].

It is not easy to define QOL in single sentence QOL is such a broad domain with lot of subjective perceptions. Many researchers have tried to give one definition of QOL and tried to make it more objective & measurable but neither of definition could explain QOL completely. Nevertheless QOL has been defined by various researchers/ organizations differently. Some of the definitions may be accessed by referring the available literature [6].

5. Various dimensions of quality of life

Broadly dimensions of QOL may be explained as Physical, Mental, Social and Functional Health. These dimensions of QOL have certain components so that every

Treatment decision making	Quality of life considerations can often be important in selecting between two or more treatment options.
Preparing for treatment experience	Information about how treatment affects quality of life can help patients prepare for and help them cope with the treatment experience
Identifying and prioritizing problems	If patients have multiple problems, quality of life reporting may help their providers to identify which are the most significant.
Facilitating communication	Quality of life measures may help patients communicate problems to healthcare providers and help staff focus on concerns that are most important to patients
Screening for hidden problems	Quality of life information can help identify problems such as depression or sexual dysfunction that may otherwise be overlooked.
Facilitating shared clinical decision making	Quality of life measures can identify patient goals, outcomes, and expectations; healthcare providers can address whether treatment is likely to meet patient expectations and discuss discrepancies between probable outcomes and patient expectations
Monitoring changes or responses to treatment	Quality of life information can help determine whether treatment is leading to improvements that are relevant to patients.

Source: [4].

Table 1.
Uses for quality of life information/measures in medical practice.

Dimensions of QOL	Components
Physical health	Somatic sensations, disease symptoms, treatment side effects/Adverse effetcs
Mental health	May vary from a positive sense of well-being to non-pathological forms of psychological distress to diagnosable psychiatric disorder/disease.
Social health	Quantitative and qualitative aspects of social contacts and interactions with each other & their assessment
Functional health	Physical functioning like self-care, mobility, and physical activity level and social role functioning in relation to family and in relation to working.

Source: [6].

Table 2.
Dimension of QOL and their respective components.

dimension may be attained more objectively. **Table 2** mentions each dimension of QOL along with their respective components. Every cancer patient should be subjected to attain all these dimensions in all possible manners [6].

6. Quality of life among cancer patients

Cancer patients tend to experience a variety of signs & symptoms. Inadequate & Improper medical management of these symptoms does hamper the performance of the day today functioning of a cancer patient including disturbed quality of life. Effective management of these symptoms will surely help in relieving the suffering from dreaded cancer and improve the quality of life (QOL) either.

These Symptoms led to major impact on QOL among the patients with breast cancers as well. This high symptom load has always been associated with the more levels of emotional suffering, poor physical & societal functioning and deteriorated QOL. Hence, effective clinical management of these symptoms can improve the QOL in cancer patients [7].

A study from India showed that cancer patients were in the below average category of QOL and the QOL of the cancer patients was influenced by reported symptoms. Very low-level QOL was observed in general, physical, psychological well-being of cancer patients. They were also suffered with below average economic well-being, pain, sleep problems and fatigue.The psychological health was affected by feeling very much depressed and they were not feeling comfortable in attending the social functions [7].

7. Parameters of quality of life

Various literatures have also explained various parameters of QOL. All treating doctors must ensure that patient to attain as many parameters as possible. Following parameters may be considered to ensure and measure quality of life among cancer patients (**Table 3**) [7].

8. Scales for QOL

Health-related quality of life is a subjective state of cancer patients and therefore must be reported or rated by individuals (patients) themselves. This QOL rating is usually done using a questionnaire. Individuals are asked to answer one or more questions in a variety of areas that include physical, emotional, and social health [8].

Physical Health: Physical functioning, satisfaction with physical ability, mobility, pain effects, pain severity, role limitations due to physical health.

1. Psychological well-being
2. General well-being
3. Physical well-being
4. Familial relationship
5. Sexual and personal ability
6. Cognitive well-being
7. Optimism and belief
8. Economic well-being
9. Informational support
10. Patient–physician relationship
11. Body image

Table 3.
Parameters for ensure and measure quality of life among cancer patients.

Mental Health: Psychological distress (anxiety and depression), psychological well-being (positive affect and feelings of belonging), cognitive functioning, role limitations due to emotional problems.

General Health: Energy/fatigue, sleep problems, psychophysiologic symptoms, social functioning, role functioning (e.g., unable to work), current health perceptions, and health distress.

Some of the scales are also available to measure the QOL among cancer patients as mentioned below [8]:

1. Functional Assessment of Cancer Therapy (FACT) scale for breast cancer (FACT-B)

2. Memorial Symptom Assessment Scale (MSAS)

3. European Quality of Life-5D (EQ-5D)

4. Kornblith Fear of Recurrence Scale

5. Decision-Making and Risk-Benefit Evaluation

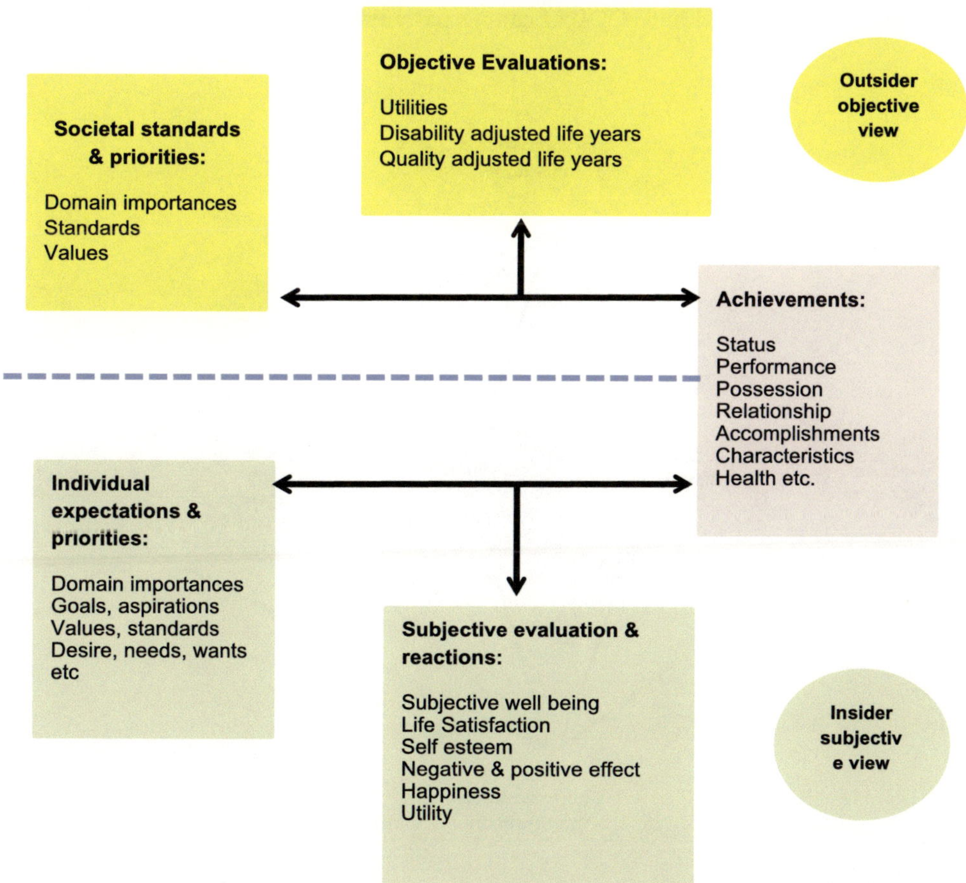

Figure 1.
Source: [9].

9. Models of quality of life

Various models have also been suggested for assessment of QOL among patients including cancer patients. Following are the various models of QOL:

1. Dijkers's model of quality of life and its evaluation (**Figure 1**)

2. Wilson and Cleary model of quality of life (**Figure 2**)

3. PROMIS conceptual model (**Table 4**)

4. Function-Neutral Health-Related Quality of Life Measure (**Table 5**)

10. Impact of screening of Cancer disease & QOL of cancer patients

Screening will ensure early diagnosis among cancer patients. Early diagnosis and treatment gives sense of confidence among cancer patients that they may either be cured or if not, may have good survival probability. This all psychological effects of screening will surely add in to QOL of cancer patients [1].

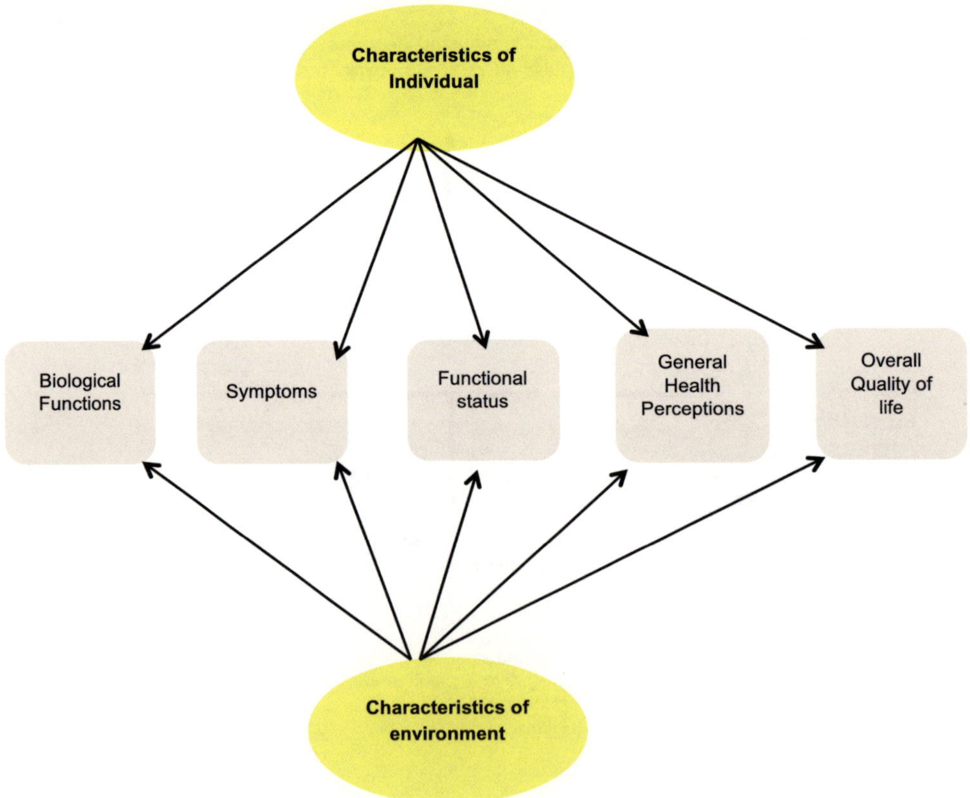

Figure 2.
Source: [10].

	Physical Health	Mental Health	Social Health
PROMIS Profile domains	Physical health Pain intensity Pain interference Fatigue Sleep disturbance	Depression Anxiety	Ability to participate in social role and responsibilities
PROMIS Additional domains	Pain behavior Pain quality Sleep related impairment Sexual functions Gastro intestinal symptoms Dyspnea	Anger Cognitive functions Alcohol use, consequences, expectancies Psychosocial illness impact Self-efficacy Smoking	Satisfaction with social roles & activities Social support Social isolation Companionship

Source: [11].

Table 4.
PROMIS conceptual model.

Health Related Quality of Life				Ancillary
Physical health	**Mental health**	**Social health**	**Life satisfaction/ Belief**	**Environment**
Energy/ fatigue Stamina Pain Sick /well Rest	Distress Affect/mood Memory Decision making Emotional regulation	Civic engagement Social engagement Relationship Intimacy Oppression/ discrimination	Livings ones values Meaning of life Life satisfaction Recreation Meaningful activities	Safety & security Access to service & transportation Public policies Societal attitudes Air /water/climate

Source: Krahn et al. [12]

Table 5.
Function-neutral health-related quality of life measure.

11. Impact of QOL on life expectancy of various cancers

Different cancers have all range of life expectancies, some of them are having very good life expectancy and some are having very less. This life expectancy is always influenced by the quality of life a cancer patient live after getting diagnosed and when on treatment. Cancer treating medical professional must never forget role of QOL in survival of cancer patients. Maintenance of good QOL should be integral part of prevention and control on all cancers. Good quality of life among cancer patients will also have an impact on DALYs (Disability adjusted life years) and this reduction of morbidity will provide opportunity to cancer patients for their social and vocational rehabilitation. This will also ensure to live most productive life among cancer patients [7].

12. QOL improvement among cancer patients

Cancer patients tend to experience array of signs & symptoms which can affect their QOL. The Medical & clinical management of cancer pain is one of most critical

& priority issue in the care & effective treatment of patients with cancer. All health & medical professionals must make sure that all cancer patients must receive education and care adequately & well on time. There is always a felt need to develop measures & policies for effective management of sign & symptoms in a bid to improve the QOL among cancer patients. Predominant issues for cancer patient's management are the adequate & effective management of symptoms and embark on policies & strategies that will empower the cancer patients to have a better sense of control & wisdom over their illness and treatment [7].

13. Conclusion

1. Cancer is one rapidly rising non communicable disease worldwide. Cancer is not only affecting patients physically but also affecting psychological, mental & social health of patients. Cumulatively, it will impact upon the quality of life of patients.

2. There are various dimensions and models of QOL which may be followed to ensure & measure QOL among patients.

3. QOL is not easy to measure, despite this many researchers have coined the definition of QOL and certain scales are also available to measure the QOL more objectively.

4. Cancer treating medical professionals must also consider this aspect of QOL along with curative treatment of cancer patients.

Author details

Neeraj Gour* and Meenakshi Chaudhary
SHKM Govt. Medical College, Nalhar, Haryana, India

*Address all correspondence to: drneerajg04@gmail.com

References

[1] Module for Multi-Purpose Workers (MPW) -on Prevention, Screening and Control of Common NonCommunicableDiseases. 2022. Available from: https://main.mohfw.gov.in/sites/default/files/Module%20for%20MultiPurpose%20Workers%20-%20Prevention%2C%20Screening%20and%20Control%20of%20Common%20NCDS_2.pdf [Accessed on 16th July 2022]

[2] Van Wilder L, Clays E, Devleesschauwer B, et al. Health-related quality of life in patients with non-communicable disease: Study protocol of a cross-sectional survey. BMJ Open. 2020;**10**:e037131. DOI: 10.1136/bmjopen-2020-037131

[3] Ferlay J, Soerjomataram I, Dikshit R, Eser S, Mathers C, Rebelo M, et al. Cancer incidence and mortality worldwide: Sources, methods and major patterns in GLOBOCAN 2012. International Journal of Cancer. 2015; **136**(5):E359-E386. DOI: 10.1002/ijc.29210

[4] Higginson IJ, Carr AJ. Using quality of life measures in the clinical setting. British Medical Journal. 2001;**322**:1297

[5] World Health Organization. The constitution of the World Health Organization. WHO Chronicle. 1947; **1**:29

[6] Post MW. Definitions of quality of life: What has happened and how to move on. Topics in Spinal Cord Injury Rehabilitation. 2014;**20**(3):167-180. DOI: 10.1310/sci2003-167

[7] Nayak MG, George A, Vidyasagar MS, Mathew S, Nayak S, Nayak BS, et al. Quality of life among cancer patients. Indian Journal of Palliative Care. 2017;**23**:445-450

[8] Quality of Life and Patient-Reported Outcomes in Cancer. 2022. Available from: https://researchadvocacy.org/ [Accessed on 16th July 2022]

[9] Dijkers MP. Quality of life of individuals with spinal cord injury: a review of conceptualization, measurement, and research findings. Journal of Rehabilitation Research and Development. 2005;**42**(3 Suppl 1): 87-110. DOI: 10.1682/jrrd.2004.08.0100. PMID: 16195966

[10] Wilson IB, Cleary PD. Linking clinical variables with health-related quality of life. A conceptual model of patient outcomes. JAMA. 1995;**273**(1): 59-65

[11] PROMIS Conceptual Framework. 2022. Available from: http://www.nihpromis.org/measures/domainframework [Accessed on 16th July 2022]

[12] Krahn GL, Horner-Johnson W, Hall TA, et al. Development and psychometric assessment of the function-neutral health-related quality of life measure. American Journal of Physical Medicine & Rehabilitation. 2014;**93**(1):60

Chapter 3

Anxiety, Depression, and Delirium in Terminally Ill Cancer Patient

Susana Villa García Ugarte
and Luis Enrique Miranda Calderón

"The truth is, once you learn how to die you learn how to live.
—Mitch Albom, Tuesdays with Morrie[1]

Abstract

Most terminally ill cancer patients present some degree of anxiety, depression, or delirium. In many cases family concerns, the prognosis of the disease, the type of treatment, and its adverse effects aggravate these emotional symptoms to the point of turning them into severe affective disorders which severely complicate their emotional state, their physical condition and their disposition and response to treatment. Although these are high prevalence disorders in terminally ill cancer patients, they often go undiagnosed and therefore do not receive treatment. An early diagnosis and adequate treatment, that includes emotional accompaniment, can greatly help to maintain the quality of life or even improve it and make these patients and their families move in a dignified way toward death. The scope of this chapter is to establish the presence of anxiety, depression and delirium in terminally ill cancer patients through scientific evidence; review the opinion of experts in the field on the most appropriate treatment, and the influence on the beneficial impact of interventions with family members or support people to ensure a more positive approach to the circumstances of these patients and serve as support for the treatment of medical personnel.

Keywords: anxiety, depression, delirium, terminally ill patient, oncology, quality of life, good death

1. Introduction

1.1 Cancer: definition and prevalence

Cancer is defined as the pathological tissue growth caused by a lengthy and persistent proliferation of abnormal cells which causes invasion and destruction of body tissues [1].

Cancer, neoplasm, or malignant tumors are generic terms used in an indistinct way to designate a wide group of diseases that can affect any part of the organism. But cancer has a definite characteristic: the accelerated multiplication of abnormal cells that extend far beyond their usual limits, even invading other body parts, which is called metastasis. The metastatic extension is the principal cause of death by the disease [2].

According to the World Health Organization (WHO), cancer is the principal cause of death worldwide, being almost one of six deaths registered annually and in 2020, the total amount of cancer-related deaths was nearly 10 million [2].

Approximately 400 thousand children get diagnosed with any type of cancer annually. However, the incidence rises with age due to the loss of cellular repair mechanisms and the accumulation of risk factors [2].

Besides age, smoking is another important cancer risk factor, being almost one-third of cancer-related deaths. Other risk factors are increased body mass index, a sedentary lifestyle, alcohol intake, and low fruit intake [2].

2. Anxiety: definition, prevalence, and clinical characteristics

Anxiety is a natural adaptive mechanism that allows the human being to be alert to potential dangers. In a way, it delivers a sense of precaution for usual dangers and, in moderate intensity and short intervals, can help us focus, maintain focus, and face challenges.

As with other emotions, when the anxiety presents disproportionately for a specific situation or even in the absence of any evident danger, the beneficial effect is exceeded.

According to WHO, in 2015 the world prevalence of anxiety disorders was 3,6%. As with depression, anxiety disorders are more frequent in women than in men (4.6% versus 2.6% worldwide) [3].

It is calculated that approximately 13% of the general population has a phobic anxiety disorder, like social phobia, whereas 7% of women and 4.3% of men have specific phobias. Generalized anxiety disorder (GAD) is presented in 3–5% of the adult population. Obsessive-compulsive disorder (OCD) affects almost 2.3% of adults. Panic disorder is less frequent and is diagnosed in less than 1% of the population. Posttraumatic stress affects at least 1% of the population, with higher incidences in war veterans and survivors of physical or sexual abuse [3].

As physical signs and symptoms, we can find palpitations, tachycardia, hyperventilation, excessive sweating, the feeling of chest oppression or dyspnoea, tremors, dizziness, and fainting. As mental signs and symptoms, we have constant worry, weariness, irritability, and trouble focusing and falling asleep [4].

The anxiety that occurs in a high level of intensity and extends for long periods begins to produce a psychosocial functioning deterioration, interfering with normal activities and in more than one sphere (social, family, academic, and work, among others). On the other hand, the intensity and duration also produce physiological damage.

It is important to promptly recognize these signs and symptoms and have an integral medical evaluation.

3. Depression: definition, prevalence, and clinical characteristics

Mental health problems, especially depression, represent a public health concern due to their high prevalence, morbimortality, and incapacity generated in a long term.

Depression is different from mood changes and brief emotional responses to the problems of daily life and can become a serious health problem, especially when it occurs recurrently and with moderate to severe intensity, being associated with suicide in some cases.

Depression is a common disease throughout the world, as it is estimated to affect 5% of adults and 5.7% of elderly adults (over 60 years of age) [5]. According to the WHO, it is estimated that, in 2015, the proportion of the world population with depression was 4,4%. Although since the start of the 2019 COVID pandemic, the prevalence of anxiety and depression has increased by up to 25% [6].

In general, depression is defined as a disease characterized by a state of persistent sadness that is accompanied by a loss of interest in previously enjoyed activities. In addition, the patient loses the ability to carry out daily activities. All of this occurs for at least two weeks. In many cases, when depression is chronic, it is difficult for the patient to identify sadness or even remember what activities generated enjoyment: the only thing noticeable is the difficulty to participate in their different spheres (social, sentimental, work, academic, etc.) [7].

People with depression often have several of the following symptoms: loss of energy, disturbances in sleep pattern, sleeping more or less than usual; changes in the appetite; anxiety; decreased concentration; indecision; concern; feeling worthless, guilty, or hopeless; and frequent thoughts related to death, with self-harm, suicidal thoughts or attempts that often lead to death [8].

People exposed to violence frequently experience a variety of reactions including anxiety, stress, frustration, fear, irritability, anger, difficulty concentrating, loss of appetite, and nightmares [9].

Depression interferes with daily life, the ability to work, sleep, study, eat and enjoy life [9]. On the other hand, people with depression present cognitive distortions, such as negative thoughts about themselves, the environment or the future, and alterations in cognitive performance such as difficulties with concentration, memory, and the ability to make decisions, which also influence the overall functioning of the person [8].

When talking about mental health, it is always important to emphasize that depression is not a sign of weakness. It can be treated with psychotherapy, antidepressant medication or with a combination of both methods, the latter being what has shown better and longer-lasting results. A second sphere that must be targeted, within the treatment, is the generation of healthy lifestyles.

It is very common for patients with depression to have a family history of the disease. However, depression can also occur in people without a family history.

The causes of depression are multiple since several genetic, biological, and environmental factors intervene in it.

Regarding genetic factors, several studies have reported that around 200 genes are related. These genetic factors are related to alterations of neurotransmitters, cytokines and hormones, whose actions induce structural and functional modifications in the central nervous system, the endocrine system, and the immune system, which increase the risk of suffering from major depression [10].

The biological causes are explained both by structural alterations in the brain as well as functional alterations in neurotransmitters (serotonin, norepinephrine, and dopamine). However, more studies are still needed to understand the mechanisms of the efficacy of antidepressants [11, 12].

Among the environmental or psychosocial factors, it has been observed that depression is associated with previous stressful events, especially when these occur at an early or older age if the subject has been subjected to prolonged stress. The stress that accompanies the first episode produces long-term changes in brain physiology that can produce variations at the structural level and in the functioning of different brain areas [13, 14].

4. Terminally ill patients

The importance of determining that a patient is in the terminal phase (end of life) of the disease is aimed at early identification of the needs and special care that help the patient and his family [15].

Thus, the terminal patient is the one who has an advanced, progressive, and incurable disease, with a lack of reasonable possibilities of responding to a specific treatment, who presents numerous problems or intense symptoms, with a loss of autonomy or progressive fragility that represent a great emotional impact for himself, his relatives and the therapeutic team that cares for him, and his situation being related, implicitly or explicitly, to the presence of death and a life expectancy of fewer than six months. All of this is associated with high demand and use of resources [16, 17].

5. Cancer patient in terminal phase

On the other hand, the cancer patient in the terminal phase is the one with a histological diagnosis of cancer demonstrated in clinical stage IV; brain, spinal cord, liver or multiple lung metastases; who have received effective standard therapy and/or are in a situation of little or no possibility of responding to active or specific treatment [18].

Medicine attempts to preserve life, we see life expectancy rates are increasingly higher, however, it is inevitable getting to prevent death in spite of the multiple human and technological efforts and the advance in science.

It is in light of this reality that medical practitioners face patients in terminal, a human being that encounters great fears—resulting from the disease itself – to face death as an imminent situation and along with the patient, relatives and friends surrounding them.

Just there is where the medical practitioner and the therapeutic team are faced to great challenges, on the hand, relieving physical symptomatology, and on the other hand, dealing with those psychological needs. Therefore, the awareness of healthcare personnel facing this critical situation is essential to effectively help in the relief of patient and their family.

According to the Institute of Medicine, the "Good death" is one that is: "free from avoidable distress and suffering for the patient, family and caregivers, in general accord with the patient's and family's wishes, and reasonably consistent with clinical, cultural, and ethical standards" [19, 20].

The objective of the health personnel who oversees the patient in palliative care must be to reach the "Good death" and the steps to get to that state are aimed at relieving the mental, physical, family state, etc. It is there that psychiatric disorders take on great importance, because, although they are very frequent and with a high incidence, many times they are not detected early [15].

6. Psychiatric disorders in cancer patients

Within the main psychiatric disorders, we focused on the most critical three, which are anxiety, depression, and delirium.

It is evident that assessing the symptoms and signs of the different psychiatric disorders is difficult in an oncological patient in a terminal state of illness, which is why it requires greater knowledge of the most frequent psychiatric pathologies, as well as the earliest possible management of the patient to achieve a better result that improves the quality of life of our patient, as well as a "good death".

As Stiefel et al. mention underdetection and undertreatment of depression is a serious problem in palliative care [21]. In palliative care patients, anxiety and depression need to be actively screened for and dealt with using a multidisciplinary approach [22].

7. Anxiety in cancer patients

It is also important to refer to specific situations that cancer patients experience, such as radiotherapy treatments, which will be an important factor in the patient's quality of life. When the patient is presented with the different types of treatments, the first reactions to the proposed treatment arise first and special attention must be paid since many patients have preconceived ideas about side effects. This is where the role of the doctor is essential to start the new therapeutic approach, clarifying doubts [23, 24].

In the case of patients undergoing radiotherapy, some degree of anxiety has been observed, expressed mainly as concern about the treatment, side effects, what is going to happen in the near future, depression and social isolation caused mainly by fear of the treatment and its side effects and impact on quality of life [23, 24].

In this chapter we focus on the cancer patient in a terminal situation, therefore, the intention of the therapeutic treatment with radiotherapy will have the objective of improving the quality of life and not a curative intention.

Most of the effects of radiation therapy on normal tissue are attributed to cytotoxicity [25].

In the terminally ill cancer patient, the approach of the health personnel and especially of the doctor must be even more global than in any other circumstance.

We must always remember that we are dealing with a patient who not only has a feeling of uncertainty, of fear of what is going to happen, who has faced the diagnosis of "cancer" and who is also now in a terminal situation, with a logical and understandable increase of their fears, concerns, denial, physical and psychic pain, fear for their loved ones, with a very large and deep mixture of feelings that translate in a large majority of patients to some degree of anxiety, depression that the sooner we diagnose, we will be able to offer the patient and their family better adherence to treatment, a better quality of life and a more dignified death.

In studies such as the one carried out by Jung-Ah Min et al., it is observed how a high level of resilience contributes to less emotional stress in hospitalized patients. Likewise, they observe the same relationship in patients with metastatic cancer. Thus, it appears that the influence of resilience is independent of and not attributed to the potential effects of a well-known variety of factors contributing to emotional stress [26].

Resilience is defined as the dynamic capacity to successfully maintain or recover a healthy mental state in the face of significant life risks or adversities [27].

In the article published by R.L. Gould et al. evidence is shown for the feasibility and acceptability of acceptance and commitment therapy (ACT), an acceptance-based behavioral therapy, with a strong evidence base in pain and a growing evidence base in mental health conditions [4].

8. Depression in cancer patients

The diagnosis of cancer is often related to emotional and mental disorders such as depression and anxiety [26].

Psychiatric disorders, mainly anxiety and depression, occur between 25 and 50% of patients with advanced cancer; however, many of these are underdiagnosed since they are considered a part of the disease's own discomfort [28].

The comorbidity between cancer and psychiatric problems can generate several complications, ranging from non-adherence to any treatment, isolation of the patient, greater symptoms and suffering, and increased complications of recovery from surgery [29].

However, making a psychopathological diagnosis of depression in cancer patients can be difficult, due to the confluence of psychological and somatic symptoms typical of neoplastic disease. The very nature of cancer generates emotional discomfort that can range from a normal adaptive reaction to the disease to the presence of a set of signs and symptoms that, depending on the intensity and psychosocial involvement of the patient, could require psychotherapeutic and psychopharmacological treatment [30].

Insomnia, and in general, sleep disorders associated with anxiety/depressive disorders are one of the most prevalent symptoms, affecting 40–60% of cancer patients. Despite the importance of adequate sleep in cell repair processes, insomnia is one of the most common symptoms and one that generates high levels of stress but often does not receive the attention it deserves when compared to other problems presented by these patients such as nausea and pain, etc. [31].

The use of antidepressants and other psychotropic drugs is necessary for the presence of feelings of worthlessness, guilt, or hopelessness associated with frequent thoughts of death, self-harm, or suicide attempts. Pharmacological treatment can also help with irritability, anger, loss of appetite, insomnia, and difficulty concentrating and making decisions [32].

9. Depression in terminally ill patients

The incidence of major depression in terminally ill patients is between 25 and 77% [33]. Treatment should be started as soon as possible, since a lapse of time is needed for the treatment to begin to take effect, and in terminally ill patients we do not have time, we must be able to early recognize the signs and symptoms of depression that allow us to start the most appropriate treatment for each patient [34].

The sign that can help physicians in diagnosing the presence of depression is when there is a poor response to pain management, despite using different treatments. In these cases, as Robert L. Fine MD points out in his article "Depression, anxiety and delirium in terminally ill patient" [33], revising the dose of analgesics and increasing it, as well as adding antidepressant treatment, has very good results.

10. Consequences of depression in cancer patients

Cancer by itself produces enough physical and emotional discomfort in those who suffer from it, as part of its own clinical picture and as a consequence of treatments.

However, the sum of psychosocial stressors and physical alterations can trigger a depressive disorder. The association between cancer and depression worsens the suffering and quality of life of patients [34].

The association between cancer and depression also reduces therapeutic adherence and increases mortality and morbidity [35]. Depression also decreases the patient's ability to cope with the disease and exacerbates the number and intensity of physical symptoms. In this way, the hospitalization time is prolonged, it can lead to suicide and the psychological burden on the family increases [34].

In a systematic review of patients with breast, lung, brain, skin, and blood cancer, mortality was 25% higher in patients with depressive symptoms and 39% higher in patients with major or minor depression, even when the known survival clinical prognostic factors are controlled [36].

It is common to find cancer patients with suicidal ideation. People with cancer are about 2 to 3 times more likely to commit suicide than the general population. This can be caused by the specific situations of each case, such as the location of the tumor, an advanced stage, the prognosis of the disease and obviously the presence of a depressive disorder that is not identified and treated in time [37].

For this reason, it is important to diagnose depression and other psychiatric disorders in oncological patients, since not treating them can seriously complicate the prognosis of the patient [37].

11. Depression assessment in cancer patients

Through this chapter, the great importance of timely detection of depression in cancer patients has been established. Achieving the correct diagnosis helps us carry out better management, not only of the symptoms caused by the oncological disease but also an adequate intervention regarding the symptoms of depression, allowing us even to achieve an intervention of some family members in the process [38].

Even though the diagnosis is clinical and the ICD 10 or DSM5 criteria can be used, it is also possible to use some evaluation questionnaires that also allow the case to be documented properly.

For more accurate detection of depression, an evaluation in which some exploratory questions are used at the beginning is recommended; if significant symptoms are detected, it is desirable to apply some specialized test that has been previously standardized [39].

The hospital anxiety and depression scale (HAD-Hospital Anxiety and Depression Scale-HADS, Zigmond and Snaith, 1983; see **Table 1**), has been the most used self-assessment instrument to detect emotional distress (anxiety and depression) in populations with physical illness. It is a short instrument (with 14 items) that has shown reliability and validity, being used both for diagnosis and for assessing the severity of the disorder and that has been adapted and validated in various populations and cultures, always showing adequate sensitivity and specificity to discriminate anxiety and depression [39].

It consists of two subscales, HADA for anxiety and HADD for depression, of seven items each with scores from 0 to 3. It includes cognitive and affective dimensions and omits somatic aspects such as loss of appetite, fatigue, insomnia, and others to avoid attributing them to depression and not to the disease itself.

Hospital Anxiety and Depression Scale questionnaire. To evaluate anxiety and depressive state of patients with physical symptoms, they were asked to attempt a questionnaire comprising 14 items. Note: Copyright © 1983. John Wiley & Sons, Inc. Zigmond AS, Snaith RP. The hospital anxiety and depression scale. Acta Psychiatr Scand. 1983 Jun;67(6):361–370.14

A. **Do you feel tense?**	B. **Are you able to enjoy yourself to the same extent as you used to?**
Almost always	I enjoy myself exactly the same as before.
Usually	I enjoy myself less pleasure than before.
Sometimes	I enjoy myself only a little compared with before.
Never	I do not enjoy myself at all.
C. Do you have the dreadful feeling that something completely terrible might happen now?	**D.** Do you laugh to the same extent as you used to?
I have a clear dreadful feeling of something terrible happening.	I laugh the same as before
I sometimes have a dreadful feeling, but the degree is not terrible.	I do not laugh like I used to
I occasionally have a dreadful feeling, but I do not lake any notice.	I definitely do not laugh as much as I used to
I never get such a feeling.	I do not laugh at all
E. Do you ever feel worried?	**F.** Are you in a good mood?
Almost always	Not at all
Usually	Not often
Sometimes, but not frequently	Sometimes
Only occasionally	Almost always
G. Can you sit peacefully and relax?	**H.** Do you feel that you have delayed thoughts and reactions?
I can	I almost always do
I usually car	I often do
I can, but not frequently	I sometimes do
Not at all	I never do
I. Do you every feel so dreadful that you feel sick in the stomach?	**J.** Have you lost interest in your appearance?
Never	Yes, clearly
Sometimes	I do not pay enough attention to my appearance
Often	I may not pay enough attention to my appearance
Very often	I give plenty of attention to my appearance
K. Do you lack peace of mind to the extent that you must constantly move around?	**L.** Are you able to look forward to the future?
Very much so	To the same degree as before
Considerably so	Somewhat less than before
Not very much	Clearly less than before

Hospital Anxiety and Depression Scale questionnaire. To evaluate anxiety and depressive state of patients with physical symptoms, they were asked to attempt a questionnaire comprising 14 items. Note: Copyright © 1983. John Wiley & Sons, Inc. Zigmond AS, Snaith RP. The hospital anxiety and depression scale. Acta Psychiatr Scand. 1983 Jun;67(6):361–370.14	
A. **Do you feel tense?**	B. **Are you able to enjoy yourself to the same extent as you used to?**
Not at all	Almost not at all
M. Do you ever get sudden anxiety attacks?	**N.** Do you enjoy good books, radio, and television programs?
Yes, very often	Yes, often
Yes, somewhat often	Sometimes
Not often	Mot often
Never	Very rarely

Table 1.
HAD-hospital anxiety and depression scale-HADS, Zigmond y Snaith, 1983.

The authors themselves recommend the original cut-off points: eight for possible cases and > 10 for probable cases in both subscales [40].

> *"The advantage of the HADS over other instruments that assess anxious and depressive symptomatology is that it does not include somatic symptoms that can be explained by cancer or its treatment. Being a brief, easy-to-apply and reliable instrument for clinical practice and research in the cancer population, it is relevant to determine the magnitude of the problem, prevention and implementation of actions for treatment" [41].*

On the other hand, the Beck Depression Inventory-II (structured by Beck, Steer and Brown, 1996; see **Appendix A**), a self-report instrument composed of 21 items developed to evaluate the symptoms corresponding to the diagnostic criteria of depressive disorders of the Manual Diagnosis and Statistics of Mental Disorders (DSM5) has also demonstrated to have good psychometric properties, being able to detect the presence of depressive symptoms with significant clinical levels, allowing to timely intervene in the comprehensive care of cancer patients to achieve a better prognosis and better quality of care [42].

12. Treatment of depressive symptoms in cancer patients

The treatment of depressive symptoms in cancer patients is not different from that of patients with depression. The recommendation is always a multidisciplinary intervention that includes the medical treatment of the underlying disease and mental health interventions (psychiatry and psychology), social work, physical therapy, and others that speed up the recovery process or delay patient deterioration [34].

Regarding mental health, pharmacological treatment is as important as individual, group, and family psychological interventions.

It is interesting to point out that in the systematic review carried out by Dwin Gayatri et al., on "Quality of life of cancer patients at palliative care units in developing countries" [43], they find that in developing countries, patients in palliative care over 65 years of age, married or ever married, with a high level of education, users of complementary or alternative medicine, who practice religious or spiritual activities, are more likely to obtain high levels of quality of life scores.

Also, they mention that spirituality and religiosity positively affect the ability of cancer patients to cope with this situation, among other things because it gives the patient greater social support and a belief system, offering a coping mechanism and influencing neuroendocrine and neuroimmunology mechanisms.

From the medical point of view, the main way of approaching depression from the somatic area is pharmacological management. There must be coordination between the medical oncologist and the psychiatrist to choose the appropriate medication based on the patient's symptom profile, tolerability and risk-benefit, with the aim of designing a strategy for each patient [34].

Selective serotonin reuptake inhibitors (SSRIs) are effective in treating depression in cancer patients. However, it is important to consider the pharmacological interactions with antineoplastic agents that can reduce their efficacy or increase their toxicity. Fluoxetine, sertraline, paroxetine, and fluvoxamine inhibit transformation through CYP450 3A4 [44].

Other drugs like citalopram, and escitalopram, are weak inhibitors, which makes them a safer choice. Dual antidepressants have also shown efficacy due to their speed of action and their usefulness in collateral symptoms, such as vasomotor symptoms and pain. Mirtazapine is very useful in symptoms such as pain, nausea, insomnia, and anxiety [34].

Regarding the psychological approach, an intervention is important from the moment the patient is diagnosed with cancer. It should not be expected that the cancer patient manifests a psychological disorder. Primary prevention helps prevent the occurrence of subsequent clinical psychopathological conditions, such as depression [44].

Individual cognitive-behavioral psychotherapy is the one that has been more studied, proving its effectiveness. Its help is based on the restructuring of the exaggerated negative beliefs that the patient has about himself, the world and the future. The objective is that the patient can have a more realistic vision, which helps him to face life in general in a healthier way [45].

On the other hand, strategies such as mindfulness, or full attention, have become highly relevant in recent years for managing stress and somatic pain. Other strategies, such as relaxation and other imagery-based therapies, have been used in successful interventions, reported in numerous publications. Music therapy has also been shown to relieve patients' pain and psychological symptoms [46].

Among the beneficial effects of these psychological interventions is the reduction of the stress impact on the body, reduction of fear of the illness, activation of the immune system, increased motivation for lifestyle changes, strengthening the "desire to live", coping with despair and evaluation and modification of the patient's beliefs regarding the disease [44].

Another important point to keep in mind is the role of family and friends as a source of social, personal, emotional, and financial support. For this reason, it is extremely important to carry out an adequate family/or social psychological approach, addressing the concerns and difficulties that arise in the family or social support group of the cancer patient [47].

Many times, family conflicts, the sadness of losing a loved one and feelings of guilt can worsen the course of the disease, while mutual supportive relationships, unity, and family skills in caring for the sick are important protective factors [47].

13. Delirium

Delirium is a complex neurocognitive and behavioral syndrome, characterized by alterations in the level of consciousness and attention, associated with cognitive and perception alterations [48]. It has an abrupt onset and a fluctuating course.

Although its presence is very frequent, it is highly underdiagnosed. In patients with oncological and terminal pathology, its frequency varies between 26 and 44% and in recent days up to 80–90% [49].

Predisposing and precipitating factors of delirium have been described that we must consider for an early diagnosis. As described by Rolfson D, a powerful model that encourages clinicians to delineate multiple predisposing factors or vulnerability aspects and also to clearly list the acute triggers [50].

As predisposing factors, we have advanced age, male, visual disturbances, dementia, depression, physical dependence, immobility, fractured femur, alcoholism, serious physical illness, and stroke [51].

As acute triggers, we have drugs, organic involvement of the central nervous system, severe acute illness; cardiac, renal, respiratory or hepatic failure, infections, metabolic disorders such as hyponatremia, hyperkalemia, hypomagnesemia, and hypoglycemia; dehydration, anemia, disseminated intravascular coagulation and major surgery [49, 51, 52].

Opioid and nonopioid psychoactive drugs have been identified as clear precipitating factors. Also, dehydration is associated with reversible delirium [53].

Knowing its high incidence, it is necessary to always have the suspicion of being faced with this pathology, even more so when there is a reversibility chance in 50% of the cases [49] and in the ones that are not reversible, symptomatic treatment can always be carried out. Hence the importance of making a correct diagnosis and a prompt treatment that help us avoid early deaths and reduce the suffering of the patient and their families.

The diagnosis is clinical, for which we have The Diagnostic and Statistical Manual of Mental Disorders, Fifth Edition (DSM 5), (DSM 5) criteria described in **Table 2** [54, 55]. A differential diagnosis must be made with depressive episodes, psychotic events, and dementias.

DSM-5
a. Disturbance in attention (i.e., reduced ability to direct, focus, sustain, and shift attention) and awareness (reduced orientation to the environment.
b. The disturbance develops over a short period of time (usually hours to a few days), represents an acute change from baseline attention and awareness, and tends to fluctuate in severity during the course of the day.
c. An additional disturbance in cognition (i.e., memory deficit, disorientation, language, visuospatial ability, or perception).
d. The disturbances in Criteria A and C are not better explained by a pre-existing, established or evolving neurocognitive disorder and do not occur in the context of a severely reduced level of arousal such as coma.
e. There is evidence from the history, physical examination or laboratory findings that the disturbance is a direct physiological consequence of another medical condition, substance intoxication or withdrawal (i.e., due to a drug of abuse or to a medication), or exposure to a toxin, or is due to multiple aetiologies).

DSM-5 Diagnosis and Statistical Manual of Mental Disorders, fifth edition.

Table 2.
DSM-5 delirium diagnosis criteria.

Once the delirium has been diagnosed, an evaluation of the causes must be initiated, provided that the patient is not in a state of agony. All tests must be consistent with the patient's clinical status and with the expected benefit of their practice [48, 49, 56].

Among the complementary tests to request we have hemogram, coagulation, blood biochemistry (ions), kidney function, liver function, urine sediment and culture, oxygen saturation, chest X-ray, and brain CT [57].

Regarding the pathophysiology of delirium, we know that there is a wide range of causes, ranging from pharmacological to alteration of cerebral metabolism [57].

Pharmacological as a consequence of exceeding the therapeutic margin, especially with those with anticholinergic action. Opioids can cause delirium by increasing dopamine and glutamate activity and decreasing acetylcholine activity. Corticosteroids have been related to the appearance of delirium due to alteration of the hypothalamic-pituitary-adrenal axis. The neurotransmitter Gamma-aminobutyric acid (GABA), activity is decreased in delirium due to benzodiazepine and alcohol deprivation, while in hepatic encephalopathy its levels are increased by the increase in ammonia that induces the elevation of glutamate and glutamine [58, 59].

Alteration of cerebral metabolism due to a deficiency of the substances required to maintain it (mainly glucose and oxygen), toxins, or excessive metabolic demand as occurs in fever.

Likewise, cytokines also seem to be involved in the appearance of some types of delirium.

Lesions on diffuse structures composed of the thalamus and bilateral hemispheric pathways have been related to the appearance of delirium. Other structures composed of the frontal and parietal cortex of the right hemisphere and damaged by infarction of the middle cerebral artery and the right cerebral artery have also been related [60, 61].

- Hypoglycemia and hypoxemia also reduce acetylcholine [49, 53].
- Decrease or increase in brain serotonin levels.
- Infections.
- Serotonin syndrome and hepatic encephalopathy.

14. Clinical manifestations of delirium

Three types of delirium have been established according to their clinical manifestations: hyperactive, hypoactive, and mixed [51, 62].

We must take special care when facing a hypoactive type of delirium, since it is often difficult to diagnose, leading to a misdiagnosis and thus inadequate treatment.

The consciousness alteration usually fluctuates throughout the day. Alertness can be both increased and decreased. There is an attention deficit, the patient does not usually follow the dialog and responds with answers that do not correspond to the questions. The thinking process is usually incoherent or disorganized. It can also be accompanied by a language disorder that can range from dysarthria to mutism: the patient has difficulty finding the right word (dysnomia) or confuses some words with others (paraphasias). There is an alteration in immediate, short-term, or long-term memory. Disorientation, paranoid ideas, or hallucinations can also be present. The sleep-wake cycle is also usually altered. The patient may manifest an increase in pain with increases in analgesic requirements, and constructive visual apraxia (inability to copy geometric figures or more complex drawings) [49, 51, 56].

The hyperactive type predominates a psychomotor agitation, hallucinations, delusions, and a state of hyperalertness and agitation. While in the hypoactive type, a state of hypoalertness, lethargy, drowsiness, decay, and bradypsychia predominates. The mixed type is the most frequent, representing 66% of cases, characterized by alternating periods of lethargy and agitation [51, 56].

15. Treatment of delirium

Nonpharmacological measures are essential. With the environment, education and support should be carried out with the family group and close friends. Sleep hygiene, restoration of circadian rhythms, adequate environment with natural light, reducing extreme light, acoustic or thermal stimuli; avoiding if possible or at least minimizing any physical, manual or mechanical restriction, hearing and visual aids. Facilitate reorientation, transmit security and confidence to both family members and patients [57].

Neuroleptics are the drugs of choice and among them, haloperidol is the most used: it can be administered orally, intravenously, intramuscularly, and subcutaneously. Low doses of haloperidol 1–10 mg/day may usually be necessary. If it is started by the subcutaneous route, it can be started with a dose of 1.5–2.5 mg every 8 hours. It is necessary to schedule a rescue dose of 1.5–2 mg subcutaneous every 20–30 minutes. If necessary, at least 3 rescue doses can be used before switching to another, more sedating neuroleptic [49, 56, 57].

Chlorpromazine has a greater anticholinergic and sedative effect than haloperidol. However, its use is avoided subcutaneously because it is very irritating. It starts with a dose of 12.5 mg PO, IV, and IM every 4–12 hours. The same rescue dose can be used every 15–20 minutes up to a maximum of three doses before considering the use of a benzodiazepine [49, 56].

Levomepromazine has a greater sedative effect than chlorpromazine and can be indicated when the use of the subcutaneous route is needed and haloperidol is ineffective. It begins with doses of 12.5 mg PO, IM, IV, and SC every 4–12 hours, with rescue doses of 12.5–25 mg every 15–20 minutes [49, 56].

Olanzapine is an atypical neuroleptic with anxiolytic and sedative effects. The initial dose is 2.5–10 mg every 12 hours.

Risperidone is another atypical neuroleptic and can be used PO in the form of tablets or orodispersible and as an oral solution. The dose ranges between 0.25–3 mg/12–24 hours.

Benzodiazepines are indicated when neuroleptics fail to control agitation, when quick deep sedation is required, and as the first choice when delirium is precipitated by alcohol withdrawal or sedatives. Midazolam is commonly used since it can be administered by any route. The initial dose is 2.5–5 mg sc/ev every 5–10 minutes followed by a continuous infusion either sc or ev [49, 56].

In refractory cases of agitation, the use of anesthetic agents such as barbiturates or propofol may become essential.

Those cases in which the underlying cause is the use of psychotropic drugs, including opioids, and dehydration have a particularly good prognosis. We must not forget that 50% of cases of delirium are reversible, so an early and accurate diagnosis is essential.

16. Conclusions

Cancer is the principal cause of death worldwide and mental health pathologies represent a public health concern due to its high prevalence, morbimortality, and long-term disability.

The three most critical psychiatric disorders in terminally ill cancer patients are anxiety, depression, and delirium. Despite their frequency, they tend to go undiagnosed and undertreated.

The comorbidity between cancer and psychiatric disorders generates several complications, ranging from non-adherence to any treatment, social isolation of the patient, greater symptoms and suffering, increased complications during recovery from surgery, high risk of disease progression and decrease of quality of life and other issues being observed in terminally ill cancer patients. We must bear in mind that 50% of all cases of delirium are reversible, so early, and accurate diagnosis is paramount.

The early detection and management of both psychic and psychological symptoms will improve patients' quality of life and good death, positively impacting not only the patients but also their caregivers.

Treatment of mental health problems in cancer patients is no different than in other patients. The recommendation is always to provide a multidisciplinary intervention that includes medical treatment of the underlying disease as well as of the mental health (psychiatry and psychology), social work support, physiotherapy and others that speed up the recovery process or delay the deterioration of the patient's health.

Psychotherapeutic interventions should also be included for family and support group to help maintaining and improving the quality of life of these patients and allow them and their families to transition to death with dignity.

Appendix A: Beck's depression inventory

This depression inventory can be self-scored. The scoring scale is at the end of the questionnaire.

1.

    0. I do not feel sad.

    1. I feel sad

    2. I am sad all the time and I can't snap out of it.

    3. I am so sad and unhappy that I can't stand it.

2.

    0. I am not particularly discouraged about the future.

    1. I feel discouraged about the future.

    2. I feel I have nothing to look forward to.

    3. I feel the future is hopeless and that things cannot improve.

3.

0. I do not feel like a failure.

1. I feel I have failed more than the average person.

2. As I look back on my life, all I can see is a lot of failures.

3. I feel I am a complete failure as a person.

4.

0. I get as much satisfaction out of things as I used to.

1. I don't enjoy things the way I used to.

2. I don't get real satisfaction out of anything anymore.

3. I am dissatisfied or bored with everything.

5.

0. I don't feel particularly guilty.

1. I feel guilty a good part of the time.

2. I feel quite guilty most of the time.

3. I feel guilty all of the time.

6.

0. I don't feel I am being punished. .

1. I feel I may be punished.

2. I expect to be punished.

3. I feel I am being punished.

7.

0. I don't feel disappointed in myself.

1. I am disappointed in myself.

2. I am disgusted with myself.

3. I hate myself.

8.

0. I don't feel I am any worse than anybody else.

1. I am critical of myself for my weaknesses or mistakes.

2. I blame myself all the time for my faults.

3. I blame myself for everything bad that happens.

9.

0. I don't have any thoughts of killing myself.

1. I have thoughts of killing myself, but I would not carry them out.

2. I would like to kill myself.

3. I would kill myself if I had the chance.

10.

0. I don't cry any more than usual.

1. I cry more now than I used to.

2. I cry all the time now.

3. I used to be able to cry, but now I can't cry even though I want to.

11.

0. I am no more irritated by things than I ever was.

1. I am slightly more irritated now than usual.

2. I am quite annoyed or irritated a good deal of the time.

3. I feel irritated all the time.

12.

0. I have not lost interest in other people.

1. I am less interested in other people than I used to be.

2. I have lost most of my interest in other people.

3. I have lost all of my interest in other people.

13.

0. I make decisions about as well as I ever could.

1. I put off making decisions more than I used to.

2. I have greater difficulty in making decisions more than I used to.

3. I can't make decisions at all anymore.

14.

0. I don't feel that I look any worse than I used to.

1. I am worried that I am looking old or unattractive.

2. I feel there are permanent changes in my appearance that make me look unattractive

3. I believe that I look ugly.

15.

0. I can work about as well as before.

1. It takes an extra effort to get started at doing something.

2. I have to push myself very hard to do anything.

3. I can't do any work at all.

16.

0. I can sleep as well as usual.

1. I don't sleep as well as I used to.

2. I wake up 1–2 hours earlier than usual and find it hard to get back to sleep.

3. I wake up several hours earlier than I used to and cannot get back to sleep.

17.

0. I don't get more tired than usual.

1. I get tired more easily than I used to.

2. I get tired from doing almost anything.

3. I am too tired to do anything.

18.

0. My appetite is no worse than usual.

1. My appetite is not as good as it used to be.

2. My appetite is much worse now.

3. I have no appetite at all anymore.

19.

0. I haven't lost much weight, if any, lately.

1. I have lost more than five pounds.

2. I have lost more than ten pounds.

3. I have lost more than fifteen pounds.

20.

0. I am no more worried about my health than usual.

1. I am worried about physical problems like aches, pains, upset stomach, or constipation.

2. I am very worried about physical problems and it's hard to think of much else.

3. I am so worried about my physical problems that I cannot think of anything else.

21.

0. I have not noticed any recent change in my interest in sex.

1. I am less interested in sex than I used to be.

2. I have almost no interest in sex.

3. I have lost interest in sex completely.

Interpreting the beck depression inventory

Now that you have completed the questionnaire, add up the score for each of the twenty-one questions by counting the number to the right of each question you marked. The highest possible total for the whole test would be sixty-three. This would mean you circled number three on all twenty-one questions. Since the lowest possible score for each question is zero, the lowest possible score for the test would be zero. This would mean you circles zero on each question. You can evaluate your depression according to the Table below.

Total score	Levels of depression
1–10	These ups and downs are considered normal
11–16	Mild mood disturbance
17–20	Borderline clinical depression
21–30	Moderate depression
31–40	Severe depression over
40	Extreme depression

http://www.med.navy.mil/sites/NMCP2/PatientServices/SleepClinicLab/Documents/Beck_Depression_Inventory.pdf

Author details

Susana Villa García Ugarte[1*] and Luis Enrique Miranda Calderón[2]

1 Family Doctor, Servicio Madrileño de Salud, Spain

2 Psychiatrist and Psychotherapist, Member of the Unidad de Salud, Cuidados Paliativos y Duelo en CONOSER Psicólogos and Salud Mental, Peru

*Address all correspondence to: susana_villagarcia@hotmail.com

References

[1] Guerrero J, Prepo A, Loyo J. Autotrascendencia, ansiedad y depresión en pacientes con cáncer en tratamiento. Revista Habanera de Ciencias Médicas. 2016;**15**(2):297-309

[2] Ferlay J, Ervik M, Lam F, Colombet M, Mery L, Piñeros M, et al. Global Cancer Observatory: Cancer Today. Lyon: International Agency for Research on Cancer; 2020

[3] World Health Organization. Depression and other common mental disorders: global health estimates. No. WHO/MSD/MER/2017.2. World Health Organization; 2017

[4] Gould RL, Wetherell JL, Kimona K, Serfaty MA, Jones R, Graham CD, et al. Acceptance and commitment therapy for late-life treatment-resistant generalized anxiety disorder: A feasibility study. Age Aging. 2021;**50**(5): 1751-1761

[5] Instituto de Sanimetría y Evaluación Sanitaria. Global Health Data Exchange (GHDx). Available from: http://ghdx.healthdata.org/gbd-results-tool?params=gbd-api-2019-permalink/d780dffbe8a381b25e1416884959e88b (consultado el 1 de mayo de 2021)

[6] World Health Organization. Mental Health and COVID-19: Early Evidence of the Pandemic's Impact: Scientific Brief, 2 March 2022. CC BY-NC-SA 3.0 IGO

[7] Baena ZA, Sandoval VMA y colectivo de autores: Los trastornos del estado de ánimo. Vol. 6. no. 11. México: Revista Digital Universitaria; 2005

[8] Gonda X, Pompili M, Serafini G, Carvalho AF, Rihmer Z, Dome P. The role of cognitive dysfunction in the symptoms and remission from depression. Annals of General Psychiatry. 2015;**14**:27

[9] Gerber PD, Barrett JE, Barrett JA, Oxman TE, Manheimer E, Smith R, et al. The relationship of presenting physical complaints to depressive symptoms in primary care patients. Journal of General Internal Medicine. 1992;**7**(2):170-173

[10] Bosker FJ, Hartman CA, Nolte IM, Prins BP, Terpstra P, Posthuma D, et al. Poor replication of candidate genes for major depressive disorder using genome-wide association data. Molecular Psychiatry. 2011;**16**:516-532

[11] Bunney WE Jr, Davis JM. Norepinephrine in depressive reactions. A review. Archives of General Psychiatry. 1965;**13**:483-494

[12] Schildkraut J. The catecholamine hypothesis of affective disorders: A review of supporting evidence. The American Journal of Psychiatry. 1965; **122**:509-522

[13] Racagni G, Popoli M. Cellular and molecular mechanisms in the long-term action of antidepressants. Dialogues in Clinical Neuroscience. 2008;**10**(4):385-400

[14] Gilbertson MW, Shenton ME, Ciszewski A, Kasai K, Lasko NB, Orr SP, et al. Smaller hippocampal volume predicts pathologic vulnerability to psychological trauma. Nature Neuroscience. 2002;**5**:1242-1247

[15] Rome RB, Luminais HH, Bourgeois DA, Blais CM. The role of palliative care at the end of life. The Ochsner Journal. Winter. 2011;**11**(4): 348-352

[16] Padrón Chacón R. El paciente en estado terminal. Revista Bioética. 2008; **8**(2):15-19

[17] Amado, José y Oscanoa, Teodoro. Definiciones, criterios diagnósticos y valoración de la terminalidad en enfermedades crónicas oncológicas y no oncológicas. Horizonte Médico (Lima). 2020;**20**(3):e1279. DOI: 10.24265/horizmed.2020.v20n3.11

[18] Sociedad Española de Cuidados Paliativos (SECPAL). Guía de Cuados Paliativos. 2014:1-51

[19] Field MJ, Cassel CK, editors. Approaching Death: Improving Care at the End of Life. Washington, DC: National Academy Press; 1997

[20] Kehl KA. Moving toward peace: an analysis of the concept of a good death. The American Journal of Hospice & Palliative Care. 2006;**23**(4):277-286

[21] Stiefel F, Trill M, Berney A, et al. Depression in palliative care: A pragmatic report from the Expert Working Group of the European Association for Palliative Care. Support Care Cancer. 2001;**9**:477-488

[22] Bužgová R, Jarošová D, Hajnová E. Assessing anxiety and depression with respect to the quality of life in cancer inpatients receiving palliative care. European Journal of Oncology Nursing. 2015;**19**(6):667-672

[23] Seol KH, Bong SH, Kang DH, Kim JW. Factors associated with the quality of life of patients with cancer undergoing radiotherapy. Psychiatry Investigation. 2021;**18**(1):80-87

[24] Peck A, Boland J. Emotional reactions to radiation treatment. Cancer. 1977;**40**(1):180-184

[25] Prise KM, Schettino G, Folkard M, Held KD. New insights on cell death from radiation exposure. The Lancet Oncology. 2005;**6**(7):520-528

[26] Min JA, Yoon S, Lee CU, Chae JH, Lee C, Song KY, et al. Psychological resilience contributes to low emotional distress in cancer patients. Supportive Care in Cancer. 2013; **21**(9):2469-2476

[27] Wu G, Feder A, Cohen H, Kim JJ, Calderon S, Charney DS, et al. Understanding resilience. Frontiers in Behavioral Neuroscience. 2013;**7**:10

[28] Sanna P, Bruera E. Insomnia and sleep disturbances. European Journal of Palliative Care. 2002;**9**(1):8-12

[29] Berrospi-Reyna S, Herencia-Souza M, Soto A. Prevalencia y factores asociados a la sintomatología depresiva en mujeres con cáncer de mama en un hospital público de Lima. Acta Médica Peruana. 2017;**34**(2):95-100

[30] Angelino AF, Treisman GJ. Major depression and demoralization in Cancer patients: diagnostic and treatment considerations. Support Care Cancer. 2001;**9**:344-349

[31] Portenoy RK, Itri IM. Cancer-related fatigue: guidelines for evaluation and management. The Oncologist. 1999;**4**(1): 1-10

[32] Ballenger JC, Davidson TRT, Lecrubier Y, Nutt DJ, Jones RD, Berard RMF. Consensus Statement on Depression, Anxiety, and Oncology. The Journal of Clinical Psychiatry. 2001;**62** (Suppl. 8):64-67

[33] Fine RL. Depression, anxiety, and delirium in the Terminally Ill patient. Baylor University Medical Center Proceedings. 2001;**14**(2):130-133

[34] García PB, Algar MJM. Tratamiento farmacológico de la depresión en cáncer. Psicooncología. 2017;**13**(2–3):249-270

[35] Teng CT, De Castro H. y Navas FD. Depressão e comorbidades clínicas. Revista de Psiquiatría Clínica. 2005; **32**(3):149–159

[36] Barber B, Dergousoff J, Slater L, Harris J, O'Connell D, El-Hakim H, et al. Depression and survival in patients with head and neck cancer: A systematic review. JAMA Otolaryngology: Head & Neck Surgery. 2016;**142**(3):284–288

[37] Hernández M, Cruzado JA, Prado C, Rodríguez E, Hernández C, González MA, y Martín JC. Salud mental y malestar emocional en pacientes con cáncer. Psicooncología. 2012;**9**(2-3):233-257

[38] Landa-Ramírez E, Cárdenas-López G, Greer JA, Sánchez-Román S, Riveros-Rosas A. Evaluación de la depresión en pacientes con cáncer terminal y su aplicación en el contexto mexicano: Una revisión. Salud Mental. 2014;**37**(5):415-422

[39] Rivera J, Alegre C, Ballina F, Carbonell J, Carmona L, Castel B, et al. Documento de consenso de la Sociedad Española de Reumatología sobre la fibromialgia. Reumatología Clínica. 2006;**2**:55-66

[40] Zigmond A, Snaith R. The hospital anxiety and depression scale. Acta Psychiatrica Scandinavica. 1983;**67**: 361-370

[41] Galindo Vázquez O, Benjet C, Juárez García F, Rojas Castillo E, Riveros Rosas A, Aguilar Ponce JL, et al. Propiedades psicométricas de la Escala Hospitalaria de Ansiedad y Depresión (HADS) en una población de pacientes oncológicos mexicanos. Salud Mental. 2015;**38**(4):253-258

[42] Vázquez ÓG, Castillo ER, García AM, Ponce JLA, Aguilar SA. Propiedades psicométricas del Inventario de Depresión de Beck II en pacientes con cáncer. Psicología y Salud. 2016;**26**(1): 43-49

[43] Gayatri D, Efremov L, Kantelhardt EJ, Mikolajczyk R. Quality of life of cancer patients at palliative care units in developing countries: Systematic review of the published literature. Quality of Life Research. 2021;**30**(2): 315-343

[44] Rodríguez VP, Amboage AM, Blázquez MH, Torres MÁG, Gaviria M. Depresión y cáncer: Una revisión orientada a la práctica clínica. Revista Colombiana de Cancerología. 2015; **19**(3):166-172

[45] Galindo-Vázquez O, Pérez-Barrientos H, Alvarado-Aguilar S, Rojas-Castillo E, Ángel Álvarez-Avitia M. y Aguilar-Ponce J. Efectos de la terapia cognitivo conductual en el paciente oncológico: Una revisión. Gaceta Mexicana de Oncología. 2013; **12**(2):108–115

[46] Gao Y, Wei Y, Yang W, Jiang L, Li X, Ding J, et al. The effectiveness of music therapy for terminally Ill patients: A meta-analysis and systematic review. Journal of Pain and Symptom Management. 2019;**57**(2):319-329

[47] Fuchs-Tarlovsky V, Bejarano M, Álvarez K, Godoy M, Fernández NC. Efecto de la presencia de los familiares sobre la depresión en mujeres hospitalizadas con cáncer. Revista Venezolana de Oncología. 2013;**25**(2): 190-195

[48] Fuentes C, Schonffeldt M, Rojas O, Briganti M, Droguett M, Muñoz E, et al. Delirium en el Paciente Oncológico. Revista Médica Clinica Las Condes. 2017; **28**(6):855-865

[49] Porta J, Serrano G, González J, Sánchez D, Tuca A, Gómez-batiste X. Delirium en cuidados paliativos oncológicos: revisión. Psicooncología. 2004;**1**(2):113-130

[50] Rolfson D. The causes of delirium. Delirium in old age. 2002;(2002): 101-122

[51] Burns A, Gallagley A, Byrne J. Delirium. Journal of Neurology, Neurosurgery, and Psychiatry. 2004; **75**(3):362-367

[52] Wilson JE, Mart MF, Cunningham C, et al. Delirium. Nature Reviews: Disease Primers. 2020;**6**:90

[53] Lawlor PG, Gagnon B, Mancini IL, Pereira JL, Hanson J, Suarez-Almazor ME, et al. Occurrence, causes, and outcome of delirium in patients with advanced cancer: A prospective study. Archives of Internal Medicine. 2000; **160**(6):786-794

[54] American Psychiatric Association: Diagnostic and Statistical. Manual of Mental Disorders, Fifth Edition. Arlington, VA: American Psychiatric Association;

[55] European Delirium Association; American Delirium Society. The DSM-5 criteria, level of arousal and delirium diagnosis: inclusiveness is safer. BMC Medicine. 2014;**12**:141

[56] Porta J, Gómez X, Tuca A. Manual de control de síntomas en pacientes con cáncer avanzado y terminal. Tercera edición. España: Instituto Catalán de Oncología; 2013

[57] Bush SH, Tierney S, Lawlor PG. Clinical Assessment ansd Management of Delirium in the Palliative Care Setting. Drugs. 2017; **77**(15):1623-1643

[58] Kaplan NM, Palmer BF. Etiology and management of delirium. The American Journal of the Medical Sciences. 2003; **325**:20-30

[59] Chan D, Brennan NJ. Delirium: making the diagnosis, improving the prognosis. Geriatrics. 1999;**54**(3):28, 36, 39-30, 36, 42

[60] Filley CM. The neuroanatomy of attention. Seminars in Speech and Language. 2002;**23**(2):89-98

[61] Schmidley JW, Messing RO. Agitated confusional states in patients with right hemisphere infarctions. Stroke. 1984;**15**(5):883-885

[62] Lipowski ZJ. Delirium (acute confusional states). Journal of the American Medical Association. 1987; **258**(13):1789-1792

Section 2

Supportive and Palliative Care in Oncology Field

Chapter 4

Palliative Care for Patients with Lung Cancer: A Review of the Current Developments in the Field and Perspectives on the Implementation of Care

Yuk-Chiu Yip, Ka-Huen Yip and Wai-King Tsui

Abstract

This chapter aims to explore the key developments in palliative care for patients with lung cancer. Lung cancer has high morbidity and mortality rates and is a leading cause of cancer-related death in the United States. Substantial evidence supports the adoption of a palliative care approach for patients with lung cancer. Palliative care aims at preventing and relieving suffering by identifying and treating debilitating symptoms early, supporting patients and their relatives to optimize coping and active living, and addressing any physical, psychosocial, and spiritual problems. An increasing number of studies show that introducing palliative care at an early stage can be beneficial for patients with advanced malignancies, including advanced lung cancer. Currently, newer palliative care approaches are being adopted, including multidisciplinary clinics and home- or community-based care. Furthermore, alternative care delivery models, such as telephone and telehealth-based approaches and outpatient palliative care, are becoming increasingly popular. However, further research is required to determine the best palliative care approach for patients with lung cancer. This chapter is a valuable contribution for both researchers and clinicians in this field, providing a more profound understanding of the existing findings in many key areas, from the developmental milestones to the adoption of holistic approaches in palliative care services for patients with lung cancer.

Keywords: lung cancer, palliative services, palliative interventions, service models, holistic care, symptom management, models of delivery, candidates for referral

1. Introduction

As a discipline, palliative care (PC) has developed rapidly since the launch of the pioneering hospice movement by Dame Cicely Saunders in the 1960s. It has become inextricably connected to optimal care for patients with serious illnesses and is now widely considered a key component of oncologic therapy in patients with advanced tumors. Moreover, it is widely agreed that patients with advanced malignancies should be referred to a PC physician at the earliest possible instance [1]. Many studies have shown that PC can improve the quality of life (QoL) of patients and their families and caregivers [2, 3].

Lung cancer is associated with high mortality and morbidity rates. It is the leading cause of cancer-related deaths in the United States, accounting for 25.9% of all cancer-related deaths in 2017 [4]. Currently, the anticipated 5-year survival rate for patients with lung cancer is only 18.1%. Even for patients with stage 1 non-small cell lung cancer (NSCLC), the 5-year overall survival rate is 73–90%, while for those with stage 4 NSCLC, it is a dismal 0–10% [5]. A meta-analysis including more than 5,000 patients with lung cancer showed that the average survival time of patients who do not undergo antineoplastic treatment is approximately 7 months [6]. Although lung cancer incidence and mortality are now declining, its prevalence remains high, with more than 500,000 people in the United States currently living with the disease [7]. For patients with advanced lung cancer, the burden of the disease, its consequences, and treatment side effects can dramatically reduce the QoL.

Lung cancer can take various forms, ranging from a silent or minimally symptomatic illness with a low burden and/or moderate progression to an aggressive and fast-progressing disease with severe symptoms. Survival rates and QoL tend to be worse in patients with advanced lung cancer experiencing severe symptoms [8]. Lung cancer symptoms include pain, nausea, dyspnea, fatigue, anorexia/cachexia, depression, and confusion/delirium [9]. Because of the high prevalence and symptom burden of the disease, the impact of PC on patients with lung cancer has attracted great research attention in recent years.

This chapter is structured to offer readers a coherent, systematic overview of the current developments and practices in the field of PC for patients with lung cancer. It starts with a brief introduction of the concepts underpinning PC, followed by an overview of research evidence that supports the role of PC in patients with lung cancer. Next, we discuss the criteria for identifying potential candidates for PC referral and explore various PC delivery models. Finally, we examine how holistic care is provided to the patients through different interventions.

2. Defining PC

The meaning of the term PC has been widely debated among healthcare professionals and the general public. The term is frequently used interchangeably with hospice care. However, hospice care focuses specifically on end-of-life practices prioritizing patient comfort over prolonging life. Patients undergoing hospice care do not usually receive disease-modifying treatments (such as antineoplastic therapies for patients with lung cancer) designed to prolong survival. This is further complicated by the fact that, in oncology, the term "palliative" is used to describe treatments that are not intended to cure, even if the key objective of the treatment is to prolong survival.

For clarity, the WHO definition of PC is employed here [10]. The WHO defines PC as a treatment approach designed to enhance the QoL of patients suffering from long-term fatal illnesses and their families by identifying, preventing, and relieving suffering as early as possible, as well as addressing physical, psychosocial, and spiritual problems. The key features of PC include a team-based approach that provides pain and symptom relief, supports patients and their relatives to optimize coping and active living, and addresses the psychological and spiritual aspects of care. PC can be delivered at any stage during an illness and used in combination with treatments designed to cure diseases or prolong survival. Although it is in no way intended to hasten death, PC does involve recognizing that death is a normal process and must be carefully thought out in advance. Specialized PC is ideally delivered by an interdisciplinary team including healthcare providers (physicians and advanced practice providers), nurses, pharmacists, chaplains, social workers, physical therapists, and dieticians.

3. Evidence supporting the role of PC in patients with lung cancer

A growing body of evidence supports using PC in patients with lung cancer. Temel et al. (2010) performed a study on early referral to PC specialists for patients newly diagnosed with advanced NSCLC [2], which is probably the most formative study on PC to date. The findings of this study showed that patients assigned to early PC combined with routine oncologic therapy had a better QoL, lower depression levels, less aggressive end-of-life care, and a significant albeit moderate improvement in overall survival. The advantages of early PC involvement in advanced lung cancer care attracted substantial research interest after this trial.

Numerous studies have found that early PC can have a positive impact on survival and QoL. For example, in the ENABLE randomized control trial, four educational sessions were held with advanced practice nurses trained in PC over the course of a week, which was followed up with monthly phone consultations. The findings showed that patients with advanced cancer undergoing PC had improved QoL [11]. Furthermore, the survival rates were found to be improved in patients with advanced cancer who were given access to a PC specialist at an early stage with monthly follow-ups [12]. Early PC was also found to reduce caregiver depression scores and stress burden [3]. In another randomized controlled trial, medical oncology clinics were randomized into PC team consultation and monthly follow-up groups [13]. The findings indicated significant improvements in end-of-life care and patient satisfaction at the primary 3-month endpoint, as well as vast improvements in the additional QoL metrics at 4 months (secondary endpoint) [13]. A recent retrospective analysis including a large cohort of patients diagnosed with advanced lung cancer who had been referred to a PC provider following their diagnosis found that survival rates were improved (i.e., the likelihood of death was reduced) in acute care settings [14]. Notably, this positive relationship with improved survival was only evident in patients who were seen by a PC specialist more than 1 month after diagnosis (but within a year). Contrarily, a negative relationship was observed among patients who were seen within the first month. Interestingly, patients referred within a month of diagnosis were seen in inpatient settings, which indicates that such appointments may have been in the end-of-life setting. The higher chances of death in such patients may be due to poor functional status, extensive disease burden, and/or poor prognosis, which may have ultimately hastened the PC referral process.

Researchers have investigated the different components involved in a PC visit to determine the optimal ways to achieve the benefits listed above. Many different patient outcomes are impacted by a PC provider's area of focus during each appointment. For instance, outpatient PC consultations can help with symptom management, prognostic information, psychosocial support, and elucidating patients' end-of-life care objectives. A prior study revealed that patients who had more consultations focusing on coping with symptoms reported better QoL and depression scores, whereas those who had more consultations focusing on treatment decisions were less likely to receive aggressive end-of-life care. Furthermore, patients with more consultations focusing on advance care planning were more likely to relocate to a hospice [15]. Studies have also shown that early PC referral improves prognostic understanding in patients with advanced lung cancer [16].

The above evidence confirms the advantages of early PC introduction. Consequently, there has been a significant increase in the number of patients referred to PC within 1 year of diagnosis of metastatic lung cancer [17]. Nevertheless, despite the increase in the proportion of patients referred to PC from 3% in 2001 to over 30% in 2013, most patients did not receive a PC referral at all, and only one-fifth of those who did, received outpatient PC services [17]. Thus, research indicates that most people with advanced lung cancer are not able to see a PC practitioner regularly, despite the well-documented advantages of this treatment approach.

4. Candidates and timing for PC referral: meeting patients' needs within the boundary of existential challenges

According to the current American Society of Clinical Oncology (ASCO) guidelines, patients with advanced cancer (and their caregivers) should be given access to PC services within 8 weeks of diagnosis and while undergoing treatment [1]. However, in reality, such volume of referrals would rapidly overload the existing PC services and further impede care for patients living in places where access to PC is limited. Moreover, there is currently a global lack of PC providers, further hindering the service.

Many attempts have been made to determine acceptable PC referral criteria for patients with cancer [18, 19] due to the misalignment between the number of patients who are eligible for referral and the number of patients who can actually be seen. For instance, Hui et al. employed a panel of 60 experts worldwide and performed a Delphi analysis to establish the major and minor criteria for guiding outpatient PC referrals [20]. Ultimately, 11 major criteria were identified, namely, (1) severe physical symptoms; (2) severe emotional symptoms; (3) requests for hastened death by the patient; (4) spiritual or existential crisis; (5) a need for help with advance planning and decision-making; morbid complications, such as (6) spinal cord compression, (7) brain or leptomeningeal metastases, or (8) delirium; (9) referral requests by the patient; (10) the passing of 3 months since diagnosis with an expected survival time of less than 1 year; and (11) disease progression following second-line therapy [20]. Moreover, 36 minor criteria were identified in cases where 70% of experts reached an agreement. This further emphasizes the difficulty of creating a list of specific criteria.

A recent observational study examined the feasibility of applying these criteria to specific groups of patients with lung cancer [21]. In this study, the previously defined Delphi criteria were reduced to six, namely, (1) severe physical symptoms; (2) emotional symptoms; (3) brain or leptomeningeal metastases; (4) cord compression/cauda equina; (5) within 3 months of cancer diagnosis and a projected survival time of less than a year; and (6) disease progression after second-line therapy. The findings showed that 82.4% of the 28,164 patients who met the criteria for PC referral based on these indicators obtained PC referral, with a median wait time of 56 days. Thus, the findings of this feasibility study indicate that this condensed list of criteria may be effective if adopted nationally.

The current guidelines proposed by the National Comprehensive Cancer Network and the American College of Chest Physicians recommend that PC be introduced at an early stage for all patients with metastatic NSCLC [22, 23]. The ASCO also advises that PC is initiated early for patients with advanced malignancies [1]. However, there are no recommendations regarding the timing of PC referral, and few studies have explored the effect of varying time points of early referral. In the study of Bakitas et al. [12], patients with advanced cancer referred for PC at the time of diagnosis and those referred 3 months later had similar scores in the QoL, mood, or use of health-care resources evaluations. One of the many reasons for providers to delay referrals until symptoms are deemed refractory may be the absence of well-defined guidelines regarding the timing of PC referral. As a result, the time points at which referrals are made are inconsistent, and in many cases, referrals are tardy.

We propose that a compromise position be adopted, one that recognizes real-world workforce issues and the absence of clear guidelines setting out the ideal referral time point yet considers cancer staging at diagnosis, patients' prognosis, and the burden of symptoms. Assuming resources permit, patients with advanced lung cancer should be referred to the PC team within 3 months of diagnosis. This will give the team the opportunity to treat symptoms as they arise and enable the patient and team to build a relationship, which will be invaluable over time as the patient's condition deteriorates. If this is not possible, patients with a high symptom burden should be prioritized regardless of the prognosis. Other patients who should be prioritized for PC referral include those with complex psychosocial stresses, those with an estimated survival prognosis of no more than 1 year, and those with disease progression following first- or second-line treatment. In our opinion, it is critical that healthcare providers have developed primary PC skills, as they will need to fill the inevitable delay between disease diagnosis and PC referral. In particular, it is recommended that healthcare providers working with patients with lung cancer develop their primary PC skills and make efforts to ensure other members of the team are similarly skilled. Symptom assessments used in oncology practices should be standardized yet modified to meet the conditions of the practice and local resources; furthermore, these should incorporate psychosocial stress assessments that can be administered routinely. Using assessments to detect stressors early can advance referrals to case managers or social workers. Similarly, informed by assessment findings, oncology nurses and advanced nurse practitioners can hold timely consultations regarding care goals and future directives. Combined, these measures would promote communication about the care goals and support patients and caregivers in end-of-life settings.

5. Diverse models of PC delivery: existing trends and future opportunities

When patients with lung cancer are admitted to the hospital, PC is traditionally provided by consultation teams in inpatient settings [24]. As PC can largely reduce hospital expenses, fee-for-service bundled payment systems have a large influence on the development of PC delivery models [25]. Specialist consultation services and inpatient PC facilities, in which the PC team members are the primary patient caregivers, are the two most common models in hospital settings. Consequently, PC is expected to be centered in inpatient settings in the USA [26, 27]. More recent models of PC include multidisciplinary clinics [2, 28–31], home- or community-based care [32, 33], alternative delivery models (such as those that employ telephone and telehealth methods [7, 34, 35]), and outpatient PC clinics [36–38]. These newer models are favored over traditional inpatient delivery models because the focus is on the upstream incorporation of PC in outpatient settings. Additionally, the care coordination and follow-up settings are better established [39]. Some of these newer PC delivery models are discussed in depth below.

5.1 Multidisciplinary PC or oncology clinics

Although the timing of PC introduction should be based on patients' needs, it is important that assessments include factors such as the patient's prognosis, time from diagnosis to median survival age (based on cancer stage), treatment trajectory (such as first or second line of treatment), and performance status [40]. Delivering PC to patients with lung cancer at the same time as their lung cancer treatment in outpatient oncology clinic settings is a well-established delivery model that has been found to improve patient outcomes [2, 28]. Similarly, breathlessness clinics also provide a multidisciplinary integrated service that often combines respiratory, physiotherapy, occupational therapy, and PC examinations and management as a one-stop treatment paradigm. Although it is not limited to patients with lung cancer, this approach has increased the patients' mastery of breathlessness (i.e., patients' feelings of control over their respiratory condition and its impact on their QoL and function) by 16% as compared with the control group [31]. Furthermore, a systematic evaluation of 37 research articles covering 18 different breathlessness services found a substantial reduction in distress due to lower breathlessness and depression ratings compared with the control groups [41]; however, no variations in the health status or QoL could be identified. PC integration in outpatient multidisciplinary settings could be the most effective model for coordinating the care of patients with lung cancer, particularly if they are also being given disease-directed treatments like radiation or chemotherapy. Nonetheless, there is a major shortage of PC professionals, as well as a lack of capacity in outpatient cancer settings at present, and these have been reported to be significant barriers hindering the widespread implementation of such approaches [26, 42, 43].

5.2 Community-based PC

The interdisciplinary community-based care offered by registered home health or hospice agencies may have influenced the development of this approach. Previous studies have shown that this model can enhance patient satisfaction, reduce care demands in emergency departments, reduce the number of hospital days, and minimize the number of skilled nursing facility days compared to administering PC in general care settings for those with serious illnesses, including approximately 61% with advanced cancer [44]. Moreover, healthcare costs dropped by 45% due to a reduction in the use of healthcare resources. In the future, community-based PC will likely become an increasingly important PC delivery model [33]. Nonetheless, evidence supporting the use of community-based PC for patients with lung cancer is limited.

5.3 Telehealth

Patients and their families, particularly those living in rural areas, have been advised to use delivery models that involve telephone and telehealth technologies to reduce travel demands. In the ENABLE trial, telephone-based assessments were employed to facilitate the delivery of PC in a rural population of patients with advanced cancer, and the results demonstrated improved QoL [2, 45]. Another study found that a nurse-led, completely telephone-based PC intervention for patients with lung cancer is feasible [35]. Although alternative PC delivery models will almost certainly include a combination of treatments (including telemedicine), existing evidence is limited to observational non-controlled research and a few quasi-experimental studies [46]. A more recent umbrella review revealed that there is still a lack of evidence to support the use of telemedicine techniques in PC [47].

Technological issues are a significant drawback of telehealth approaches, particularly when live video platforms are used. Commonly reported issues include poor connectivity and connection, slow video feed, or problems with understanding how to use the technology (particularly among older patients) [48]. These issues are more prominent among patients from lower socioeconomic groups, non-Caucasians, and those living in rural areas. Moreover, clinicians have reported that the most severely ill patients gained the least benefits from the telehealth symptom management options [49]. Thus, there is a significant research gap regarding the intersection of PC and telehealth. Nonetheless, several well-established innovative PC delivery models have been developed for patients with lung cancer. Inpatient delivery models are preferable for such patients due to the symptom burden and their frequent inpatient clinical encounters. However, research has shown that outpatient models also enable early PC integration and enhance patient outcomes. Thus, combined delivery methods based on available resources and context are critical in providing timely PC based on the guidelines proposed by the ASCO, which recommend that PC is initiated within 8 weeks of diagnosis of advanced lung cancer [1].

Based on the above, further research is required to determine the optimal methods for delivering PC to patients with advanced malignancies. The best approaches are likely to be multidisciplinary in nature and accessible to all patients in need. In order to understand the barriers hindering the universal provision of specialized PC to patients with advanced lung cancer, oncological care providers must be able to identify and address the needs of such patients as much as possible. Standard guidelines outlining the factors involved in PC (specifically in the field of oncology) have been put forward by the ASCO and the American Academy of Hospice and Palliative Medicine [50]. Experts agree that symptoms must be evaluated and managed, with a specific focus on common oncologic symptoms, such as pain, nausea, diarrhea, vomiting, and dyspnea.

6. Patient care and therapeutic interventions in PC services for patients with lung cancer

Although there are benefits to applying PC as an additional or alternative approach to improve patients' QoL even if they are not receiving cancer-directed therapy, directed treatments have been developed to alleviate disease-related symptoms, and these are discussed below.

Pain is one of the most common and debilitating symptoms in advanced malignancies. Additionally, pain tends to be a multifaceted experience of suffering that is related to psychological distress. Thus, in such cases, a multidisciplinary approach is recommended. Opioids are one of the most commonly used medicines for managing cancer-related pain, and an aggressive titration is often necessary to control pain effectively. However, given the widespread opioid abuse problem, it is important that practitioners and/or caregivers remain vigilant about any abuse/misuse while also avoiding undertreating pain. Pain caused by bone and/or liver metastases, as well as neuropathic pain, can be relieved using low-dose corticosteroids [51, 52].

Disease-related complications, including malignant effusions (pleural and pericardial) and airway obstruction, can cause dyspnea and cough in those with locally-advanced NSCLC or lung cancer metastases. Thoracentesis, pleural drain placement, and pericardiocentesis with a pericardial drain/window are examples of therapeutic procedures that can be performed for palliative reasons [53, 54]. Furthermore, methods such as bronchoscopy, photodynamic treatment, laser therapy, and stent implantation (endobronchial or vascular) can be used to ease airway obstruction [53]. Hemoptysis can be treated with arterial embolization.

Patients with advanced NSCLC, as well as those with lung metastases from other advanced cancers, may experience a sensation known as air hunger. Various pharmacologic and nonpharmacologic therapies can be considered to reduce this discomfort as much as possible. Morphine has been found to alleviate the feeling of air hunger in some people. Other opioids, such as oxycodone and fentanyl, have been examined in this context, but the findings have been conflicting [55]. A motorized fan aimed toward the face can alleviate this symptom for some individuals [56]. In such cases, benzodiazepines can also be administered as an adjuvant or a replacement for opioids to alleviate dyspnea [57].

Anticholinergic medications can be administered to minimize excessive secretions, such as scopolamine, atropine, hyoscyamine, and glycopyrrolate [58, 59]. Patients with substantial appetite and weight loss may benefit from appetite stimulants and dietary counseling. Although the effectiveness of low-dose corticosteroids in stimulating appetite is unknown [52], these drugs are often used for this purpose and as an antiemetic [51].

Fatigue is also a common symptom in those suffering from advanced-stage cancer. Other symptoms, including pain, dyspnea, and depression, can also contribute to this. Endocrinopathies and electrolyte abnormalities are potential metabolic causes that must be adequately investigated and managed. Although various medications have been studied, such as steroids, stimulants, antidepressants, and erythropoietin-stimulating agents, there is no compelling evidence for their efficacy in treating fatigue [60]. Physical activity and exercise have been found to be the most effective interventions for reducing fatigue [61].

Psychological distress and depression are common in patients with advanced cancers, particularly metastatic NSCLC. In a study examining the QoL of patients with advanced NSCLC, major depression was observed in 23% of patients and was also associated with lower median survival in this group compared with the group without depression [62]. Psychological distress has been shown to reduce the QoL, impair responsiveness to medicines, and increase hospitalization rates [63]. Dyspnea has also been found to be related to anxiety, which is often coupled with uncertainty about the course of the disease. The Hospital Anxiety and Depression Scale, Patient Health Questionnaire-4, or Generalized Anxiety Disorder 7-item scale can all be used to evaluate psychological symptoms. Two potential medications that can be used to alleviate symptoms are selective serotonin reuptake inhibitors and buspirone. The former are commonly administered to individuals with panic attacks [63], while breakthrough symptoms can be reduced using benzodiazepines. When it comes to treating anxiety, nonpharmacologic therapies are critical. Cognitive-behavioral therapy should be a key component of any therapeutic plan. Relaxation and panic control techniques, mindfulness training, distraction techniques, and breathing strategies may also be beneficial [63]. Additionally, patients suffering from social and financial stress are likely to benefit from social work engagement. Support groups can help patients connect with others experiencing similar symptoms. Moreover, the ENABLE II trial found that regular meetings with PC nurses to provide psychoeducation improved the patients' mood and QoL [11].

Spiritual distress is common among patients with a progressive life-threatening illness. Frequent concerns include questions about existence, the meaning of life, regret, and destiny. Spiritual issues may also be important to patients as they approach the end of their lives. The Spiritual Well-Being Scale or the Functional Assessment of Chronic Illness Therapy-Spiritual Well-Being can be employed to evaluate symptoms. In most cases, pharmacologic therapy is not required. Benzodiazepines or barbiturates can be used for sedative purposes in rare and refractory cases. It is important to listen to the patient's concerns actively and offer gentle reassurance, which are examples of nonpharmacologic therapies. Family involvement, pastoral care, and community and religious resources are all critical, as it can be incredibly distressing for individuals to watch a family member suffer from spiritual distress. It is thus critical to assess caregivers for exhaustion.

7. Conclusion

Despite the significant advances in the care-providing approaches for patients with lung cancer in recent years, the morbidity and mortality remain high. Cancer and its treatments can cause incredibly debilitating symptoms. PC, an approach to care for patients with life-threatening illnesses, including those with lung cancer (or any cancer), can reduce this burden. If introduced at an early stage of a patient's illness, PC can alleviate symptoms and enhance the QoL. There is even a possibility that it will increase the chances of survival. In order to provide PC timely, the ASCO guidelines recommend that it be started within 8 weeks of an advanced lung cancer diagnosis. Ideally, the patient should be referred to PC immediately after diagnosis. However, referring all patients for early PC is challenged by understaffed PC teams. Clinicians may make referrals based on their patient's burden of symptoms or psychosocial stresses. Patients with lung cancer would benefit from clinicians with primary PC skills. Therefore, clinicians should take steps to develop these skills and, from the outset, provide routine symptom and psychosocial assessments while the patient awaits the referral. To support the patient's PC needs, advanced practice providers, nurses, and social workers can be trained to provide PC through the oncology practice. Moreover, the PC approach should involve a combination of delivery methods based on available resources. A wide range of pharmacologic and nonpharmacologic tools are available to help patients manage their illnesses. Once treatment has been initiated, the patient's response should be regularly monitored. Providing appropriate holistic care will enable patients to live as long as possible with the best QoL.

Acknowledgements

This research was funded by the Institute Development Grant (IDG) of the Caritas Institute of Higher Education.

Conflict of interest

The authors declare no conflict of interest.

Author details

Yuk-Chiu Yip*, Ka-Huen Yip and Wai-King Tsui
School of Health Sciences, Caritas Institute of Higher Education, China

*Address all correspondence to: jeffreyycyip@gmail.com

References

[1] Ferrell BR, Temel JS, Temin S, Alesi ER, Balboni TA, Basch EM, et al. Integration of palliative care into standard oncology care: American Society of Clinical Oncology clinical practice guideline update. Journal of Clinical Oncology. 2017;**35**:96-112. DOI: 10.1200/JCO.2016.70.1474

[2] Temel JS, Greer JA, Muzikansky A, Gallagher ER, Admane S, Jackson VA, et al. Early palliative care for patients with metastatic non-small-cell lung cancer. The New England Journal of Medicine. 2010;**363**:733-742. DOI: 10.1056/NEJMoa1000678

[3] Dionne-Odom JN, Azuero A, Lyons KD, Hull JG, Tosteson T, Li Z, et al. Benefits of early versus delayed palliative care to informal family caregivers of patients with advanced cancer: Outcomes from the ENABLE III randomized controlled trial. Journal of Clinical Oncology. 2015;**33**:1446-1452. DOI: 10.1200/JCO.2014.58.7824

[4] National Cancer Institute. Surveillance, Epidemiology, and End Results Program. Cancer stat facts: Lung and bronchus cancer [Internet]. 2018. Available from: https://seer.cancer.gov/statfacts/html/lungb.html. [Accessed: July 13, 2022]

[5] Goldstraw P, Chansky K, Crowley J, Rami-Porta R, Asamura H, Eberhardt WE, et al. The IASLC lung cancer staging project: Proposals for revision of the TNM stage groupings in the forthcoming (eighth) edition of the TNM classification for lung cancer. Journal of Thoracic Oncology. 2016;**11**:39-51. DOI: 10.1016/j.jtho.2015.09.009

[6] Wao H, Mhaskar R, Kumar A, Miladinovic B, Djulbegovic B. Survival of patients with non-small cell lung cancer without treatment: A systematic review and meta-analysis. Systematic Reviews. 2013;**2**:10. DOI: 10.1186/2046-4053-2-10

[7] Nichols L, Saunders R, Knollmann FD. Causes of death of patients with lung cancer. Archives of Pathology & Laboratory Medicine. 2012;**136**:1552-1557. DOI: 10.5858/arpa.2011-0521-OA

[8] Mendoza TR, Kehl KL, Bamidele O, Williams LA, Shi Q, Cleeland CS, et al. Assessment of baseline symptom burden in treatment-naïve patients with lung cancer: An observational study. Supportive Care in Cancer. 2019;**27**:3439-3447. DOI: 10.1007/s00520-018-4632-0

[9] Iyer S, Roughley A, Rider A, Taylor-Stokes G. The symptom burden of non-small cell lung cancer in the USA: A real-world cross-sectional study. Supportive Care in Cancer. 2014;**22**:181-187. DOI: 10.1007/s00520-013-1959-4

[10] Sepúlveda C, Marlin A, Yoshida T, Ullrich A. Palliative care: The World Health Organization's global perspective. Journal of Pain and Symptom Management. 2002;**24**:91-96. DOI: 10.1016/s0885-3924(02)00440-2

[11] Bakitas M, Lyons KD, Hegel MT, Balan S, Brokaw FC, Seville J, et al. Effects of a palliative care intervention on clinical outcomes in patients with advanced cancer: The project ENABLE II randomized controlled trial. Journal of the American Medical Association. 2009;**302**:741-749. DOI: 10.1001/jama.2009.1198

[12] Bakitas MA, Tosteson TD, Li Z, Lyons KD, Hull JG, Li Z, et al. Early versus delayed initiation of concurrent palliative oncology care:

Patient outcomes in the ENABLE III randomized controlled trial. Journal of Clinical Oncology. 2015;**33**:1438-1445. DOI: 10.1200/JCO.2014.58.6362

[13] Zimmermann C, Swami N, Krzyzanowska M, Hannon B, Leighl N, Oza A, et al. Early palliative care for patients with advanced cancer: A cluster-randomised controlled trial. Lancet. 2014;**383**:1721-1730. DOI: 10.1016/S0140-6736(13)62416-2

[14] Sullivan DR, Chan B, Lapidus JA, Ganzini L, Hansen L, Carney PA, et al. Association of early palliative care use with survival and place of death among patients with advanced lung cancer receiving care in the Veterans Health Administration. JAMA Oncology. 2019;**5**:1702-1709. DOI: 10.1001/jamaoncol.2019.3105

[15] Hoerger M, Greer JA, Jackson VA, Park ER, Pirl WF, El-Jawahri A, et al. Defining the elements of early palliative care that are associated with patient-reported outcomes and the delivery of end-of-life care. Journal of Clinical Oncology. 2018;**36**:1096-1102. DOI: 10.1200/JCO.2017.75.6676

[16] Temel JS, Greer JA, Admane S, Gallagher ER, Jackson VA, Lynch TJ, et al. Longitudinal perceptions of prognosis and goals of therapy in patients with metastatic non-small-cell lung cancer: Results of a randomized study of early palliative care. Journal of Clinical Oncology. 2011;**29**:2319-2326. DOI: 10.1200/JCO.2010.32.4459

[17] Huo J, Hong YR, Turner K, Bian J, Grewal R, Wilkie DJ. Utilization pattern and service settings of palliative care for patients with metastatic non-small-cell lung cancer. Cancer. 2019;**125**:4481-4489. DOI: 10.1002/cncr.32478

[18] Hui D, Meng YC, Bruera S, Geng Y, Hutchins R, Mori M, et al. Referral criteria for outpatient palliative cancer care: A systematic review. The Oncologist. 2016;**21**:895-901. DOI: 10.1634/theoncologist.2016-0006

[19] Hui D, Titus A, Curtis T, Ho-Nguyen VT, Frederickson D, Wray C, et al. Implementation of the Edmonton Symptom Assessment System for symptom distress screening at a community cancer center: A pilot program. The Oncologist. 2017;**22**:995-1001. DOI: 10.1634/theoncologist.2016-0500

[20] Hui D, Mori M, Watanabe SM, Caraceni A, Strasser F, Saarto T, et al. Referral criteria for outpatient specialty palliative cancer care: An international consensus. The Lancet Oncology. 2016;**17**:e552-e559. DOI: 10.1016/S1470-2045(16)30577-0

[21] Iqbal J, Sutradhar R, Zhao H, Howell D, O'Brien MA, Seow H, et al. Operationalizing outpatient palliative care referral criteria in lung cancer patients: A population-based cohort study using health administrative data. Journal of Palliative Medicine. 2020;**23**:670-677. DOI: 10.1089/jpm.2019.0515

[22] National Comprehensive Cancer Network. Guidelines – Non-small cell lung Cancer [Internet]. 2018. Available from: https://www.nccn.org/professionals/physician_gls/pdf/nscl.pdf. [Accessed: July 17, 2017]

[23] Ford DW, Koch KA, Ray DE, Selecky PA. Palliative and end-of-life care in lung cancer: Diagnosis and management of lung cancer, 3rd ed: American College of Chest Physicians evidence-based clinical practice guidelines. Chest. 2013;**143**:e498S-e512S. DOI: 10.1378/chest.12-2367

[24] Dumanovsky T, Augustin R, Rogers M, Lettang K, Meier DE,

Morrison RS. The growth of palliative care in U.S. hospitals: A status report. Journal of Palliative Medicine. 2016;**19**: 8-15. DOI: 10.1089/jpm.2015.0351

[25] Smith TJ, Coyne P, Cassel B, Penberthy L, Hopson A, Hager MA. A high-volume specialist palliative care unit and team may reduce in-hospital end-of-life care costs. Journal of Palliative Medicine. 2003;**6**:699-705. DOI: 10.1089/109662103322515202

[26] Hui D, Elsayem A, De la Cruz M, Berger A, Zhukovsky DS, Palla S, et al. Availability and integration of palliative care at US cancer centers. Journal of the American Medical Association. 2010;**303**:1054-1061. DOI: 10.1001/jama.2010.258

[27] Morrison RS, Augustin R, Souvanna P, Meier DE. America's care of serious illness: A state-by-state report card on access to palliative care in our nation's hospitals. Journal of Palliative Medicine. 2011;**14**:1094-1096. DOI: 10.1089/jpm.2011.9634

[28] Temel JS, Greer JA, El-Jawahri A, Pirl WF, Park ER, Jackson VA, et al. Effects of early integrated palliative care in patients with lung and GI cancer: A randomized clinical trial. Journal of Clinical Oncology. 2017;**35**:834-841. DOI: 10.1200/JCO.2016.70.5046

[29] El-Jawahri A, Greer JA, Pirl WF, Park ER, Jackson VA, Back AL, et al. Effects of early integrated palliative care on caregivers of patients with lung and gastrointestinal cancer: A randomized clinical trial. The Oncologist. 2017;**22**:1528-1534. DOI: 10.1634/theoncologist.2017-0227

[30] Rabow MW, Dibble SL, Pantilat SZ, McPhee SJ. The comprehensive care team: A controlled trial of outpatient palliative medicine consultation. Archives of Internal Medicine. 2004;**164**:83-91. DOI: 10.1001/archinte.164.1.83

[31] Higginson IJ, Bausewein C, Reilly CC, Gao W, Gysels M, Dzingina M, et al. An integrated palliative and respiratory care service for patients with advanced disease and refractory breathlessness: A randomised controlled trial. The Lancet Respiratory Medicine. 2014;**2**:979-987. DOI: 10.1016/S2213-2600(14)70226-7

[32] Northouse LL, Mood DW, Schafenacker A, Kalemkerian G, Zalupski M, LoRusso P, et al. Randomized clinical trial of a brief and extensive dyadic intervention for advanced cancer patients and their family caregivers. Psycho-Oncology. 2013;**22**:555-563. DOI: 10.1002/pon.3036

[33] Kamal AH, Currow DC, Ritchie CS, Bull J, Abernethy AP. ommunity-based palliative care: The natural evolution for palliative care delivery in the U.S. Journal of Pain Symptom Management. 2013;**46**:254-264

[34] Chua IS, Zachariah F, Dale W, Feliciano J, Hanson L, Blackhall L, et al. Early integrated telehealth versus in-person palliative care for patients with advanced lung cancer: A study protocol. Journal of Palliative Medicine. 2019;**22**:7-19. DOI: 10.1089/jpm.2019.0210

[35] Reinke LF, Vig EK, Tartaglione EV, Backhus LM, Gunnink E, Au DH. Protocol and pilot testing: The feasibility and acceptability of a nurse-led telephone-based palliative care intervention for patients newly diagnosed with lung cancer. Contemporary Clinical Trials. 2018;**64**:30-34. DOI: 10.1016/j.cct.2017.11.013

[36] Meier DE, Beresford L. Outpatient clinics are a new frontier for palliative care. Journal of Palliative Medicine.

2008;**11**:823-828. DOI: 10.1089/jpm.2008.9886

[37] Rabow MW, Dahlin C, Calton B, Bischoff K, Ritchie C. New frontiers in outpatient palliative care for patients with cancer. Cancer Control. 2015;**22**:465-474. DOI: 10.1177/107327481502200412

[38] Rabow M, Kvale E, Barbour L, Cassel JB, Cohen S, Jackson V, et al. Moving upstream: A review of the evidence of the impact of outpatient palliative care. Journal of Palliative Medicine. 2013;**16**:1540-1549. DOI: 10.1089/jpm.2013.0153

[39] Pantilat SZ, Kerr KM, Billings JA, Bruno KA, O'Riordan DL. Palliative care services in California hospitals: Program prevalence and hospital characteristics. Journal of Pain and Symptom Management. 2012;**43**:39-46. DOI: 10.1016/j.jpainsymman.2011.03.021

[40] Hui D, Hannon BL, Zimmermann C, Bruera E. Improving patient and caregiver outcomes in oncology: Team-based, timely, and targeted palliative care. CA: A Cancer Journal for Clinicians. 2018;**68**:356-376. DOI: 10.3322/caac.21490

[41] Brighton LJ, Miller S, Farquhar M, Booth S, Yi D, Gao W, et al. Holistic services for people with advanced disease and chronic breathlessness: A systematic review and meta-analysis. Thorax. 2019;**74**:270-281. DOI: 10.1136/thoraxjnl-2018-211589

[42] Lupu D. American Academy of Hospice and Palliative Medicine Workforce Task Force. Estimate of current hospice and palliative medicine physician workforce shortage. Journal of Pain and Symptom Management. 2010;**40**:899-911. DOI: 10.1016/j.jpainsymman.2010.07.004

[43] Kamal AH, Bull JH, Swetz KM, Wolf SP, Shanafelt TD, Myers ER. Future of the palliative care workforce: Preview to an impending crisis. The American Journal of Medicine. 2017;**130**:113-114. DOI: 10.1016/j.amjmed.2016.08.046

[44] Brumley RD, Enguidanos S, Cherin DA. Effectiveness of a home-based palliative care program for end-of-life. Journal of Palliative Medicine. 2003;**6**:715-724. DOI: 10.1089/109662103322515220

[45] Bakitas M, Stevens M, Ahles T, Kirn M, Skalla K, Kane N, et al. Project ENABLE: A palliative care demonstration project for advanced cancer patients in three settings. Journal of Palliative Medicine. 2004;**7**:363-372. DOI: 10.1089/109662104773709530

[46] Capurro D, Cole K, Echavarría MI, Joe J, Neogi T, Turner AM. The use of social networking sites for public health practice and research: A systematic review. Journal of Medical Internet Research. 2014;**16**:e79. DOI: 10.2196/jmir.2679

[47] Rogante M, Giacomozzi C, Grigioni M, Kairy D. Telemedicine in palliative care: A review of systematic reviews. Annali dell'Istituto Superiore di Sanità. 2016;**52**:434-442. DOI: 10.4415/ANN_16_03_16

[48] Katalinic O, Young A, Doolan D. Case study: The interact home telehealth project. Journal of Telemedicine and Telecare. 2013;**19**:418-424. DOI: 10.1177/1357633X13506513

[49] Cox A, Illsley M, Knibb W, Lucas C, O'Driscoll M, Potter C, et al. The acceptability of e-technology to monitor and assess patient symptoms following palliative radiotherapy for lung cancer. Palliative Medicine. 2011;**25**:675-681. DOI: 10.1177/0269216311399489

[50] Bickel KE, Mcniff K, BussMK KA, Lupu D, Abernethy AP, et al. Defining high-quality palliative care in oncology practice: An American Society of Clinical Oncology/American Academy of Hospice and Palliative Medicine guidance statement. Journal of Oncology Practice/ American Society of Clinical Oncology. 2016;**12**:e828-e838. DOI: 10.1200/ JOP.2016.010686

[51] Shih A, Jackson KC 2nd. Role of corticosteroids in palliative care. Journal of Pain & Palliative Care Pharmacotherapy 2007;21:69-76. PMID: 18032321.

[52] Lossignol D. A little help from steroids in oncology. Journal of Translational International Medicine. 2016;**4**:52-54. DOI: 10.1515/ jtim-2016-0011

[53] Masuda E, Sista AK, Pua BB, Madoff DC. Palliative procedures in lung cancer. Seminars in Interventional Radiology. 2013;**30**:199-205. DOI: 10.1055/s-0033-1342962

[54] Farbicka P, Nowicki A. Palliative care in patients with lung cancer. Contemp Oncol (Pozn). 2013;**17**:238-245. DOI: 10.5114/wo.2013.35033

[55] Barnes H, McDonald J, Smallwood N, Manser R. Opioids for the palliation of refractory breathlessness in adults with advanced disease and terminal illness. Cochrane Database of Systematic Reviews. 2016;**3**:CD011008. DOI: 10.1002/14651858.CD011008.pub2

[56] Galbraith S, Fagan P, Perkins P, Lynch A, Booth S. Does the use of a handheld fan improve chronic dyspnea? A randomized, controlled, crossover trial. Journal of Pain and Symptom Management. 2010;**39**:831-838. DOI: 10.1016/j. jpainsymman.2009.09.024

[57] Navigante AH, Cerchietti LC, Castro MA, Lutteral MA, Cabalar ME. Midazolam as adjunct therapy to morphine in the alleviation of severe dyspnea perception in patients with advanced cancer. Journal of Pain and Symptom Management. 2006;**31**:38-47. DOI: 10.1016/j.jpainsymman.2005.06.009

[58] Wildiers H, Dhaenekint C, Demeulenaere P, Clement PM, Desmet M, Van Nuffelen R, et al. Atropine, hyoscine butylbromide, or scopolamine are equally effective for the treatment of death rattle in terminal care. Journal of Pain and Symptom Management. 2009;**38**:124-133. DOI: 10.1016/j.jpainsymman.2008.07.007

[59] Back IN, Jenkins K, Blower A, Beckhelling J. A study comparing hyoscine hydrobromide and glycopyrrolate in the treatment of death rattle. Palliative Medicine. 2001;**15**:329-336. DOI: 10.1191/026921601678320313

[60] Mucke M, Mochamat CH, Peuckmann-post V, Minton O, Stone P, et al. Pharmacological treatments for fatigue associated with palliative care: Executive summary of a Cochrane Collaboration systematic review. Journal of Cachexia Sarcopenia Muscle. 2016;**7**:23-27. DOI: 10.1002/jcsm.12101

[61] Cramp F, Byron-Daniel J. Exercise for the management of cancer-related fatigue in adults. Cochrane Database of Systematic Reviews. 2012;**11**:CD006145. DOI: 10.1002/14651858.CD006145.pub3

[62] Pirl WF, Temel JS, Billings A, Dahlin C, Jackson V, Prigerson HG, et al. Depression after diagnosis of advanced non-small cell lung cancer and survival: A pilot study. Psychosomatics. 2008;**49**:218-224. DOI: 10.1176/appi. psy.49.3.218

[63] Lanken PN, Terry PB, DeLisser HM, Fahy BF, Hansen-Flaschen J, Heffner JE,

et al. An official American Thoracic Society clinical policy statement: Palliative care for patients with respiratory diseases and critical illnesses. American Journal of Respiratory and Critical Care Medicine. 2008;**177**:912-927. DOI: 10.1164/rccm.200605-587ST

Chapter 5

Supportive and Palliative Care Attitude for Cancer Patients

Delgersuren Gelegjamts and Batbagana Burenerdene

Abstract

The purpose of this chapter is to highlight the importance of palliative care and attitude towards end-of-life among cancer patients. Besides, it will focus on how the attitude towards cancer patients is defined and structured, and what are some of the factors that can have an effect on attitude. A person's attitude towards an object (person, events, things) is determined by their feelings, emotions, beliefs, knowledge, and cultural attitudes (ethnic, racial, and religious factor). Moreover, the current chapter will try to clarify the misconceptions and fears of patients and caregivers towards palliative care and how we should try to change public perception. Attitudes towards palliative care are important not only to healthcare professionals but also to patients and their family members' attitudes toward cancer. The quality of life of a cancer patient has a direct connection with the professional and nonprofessional caregiver's knowledge of supportive care and attitude towards end-of-life care. Supportive and palliative care is an important component of the spectrum of health care services in the delivery of the best practices for cancer patients. Health care professionals play pivotal roles in the delivery of palliative care for cancer patients as they have to provide health care services with a positive attitude and also be prepared mentally.

Keywords: supportive care, palliative care, attitude, mental preparedness, end of life, cancer

1. Introduction

Recent researches have shown that a positive attitude is more beneficial to the patients than clinical treatment. The benefits include the relief of pain, improving the patient's recovery, reducing the side effects of treatment, preventing depression, Health care professionals (HCP) play an important role in improving the quality of life of patients in palliative and supportive treatment by providing them with physical, functional, emotional, and social well- and the recovery of the surgical wound is through the appropriate approach.

In order to achieve the best possible quality of life for patients and families, healthcare professionals need to acquire specific skills and have positive attitudes towards palliative care, so that they can respond appropriately to patients and their families' needs [1, 2]. HCP are not only concerned with the quality of life of the patients but also help change their attitudes towards illness, educate them on how to protect their health, and prevent different diseases. In addition, the two most important attitudes for people with cancer first is the immune level control, and second is food management. The immune level control is done by laboratory test which shows vitamins minerals deficits for you and which one is overloading in your body. Proper food management helps you to cope with your cancer, reducing the side effect of cancer treatment, preventing the spreading and the recurrence of cancer.

Therefore, the content of this topic covers are the basic concepts of attitudes, the health professionals' attitudes towards cancer patients and their families, the public attitudes towards cancer and the cancer patients' attitudes towards food and nutrition management.

2. Measurement of attitude towards palliative care

2.1 Understanding about attitude

Social-cultural knowledge is important in the understanding of palliative care [3–5]. Attitude, which referred to a force or quality of mind, seemed much more appropriate [6, 7]. Traditionally, attitudes have been considered to have three fundamental components: affective (feeling and emotional reaction) behavioral (individual intention that self-concept), and cognitive (beliefs, knowledge, thought, experience) components to the attitude object [6–9] (as shown **Figure 1**).

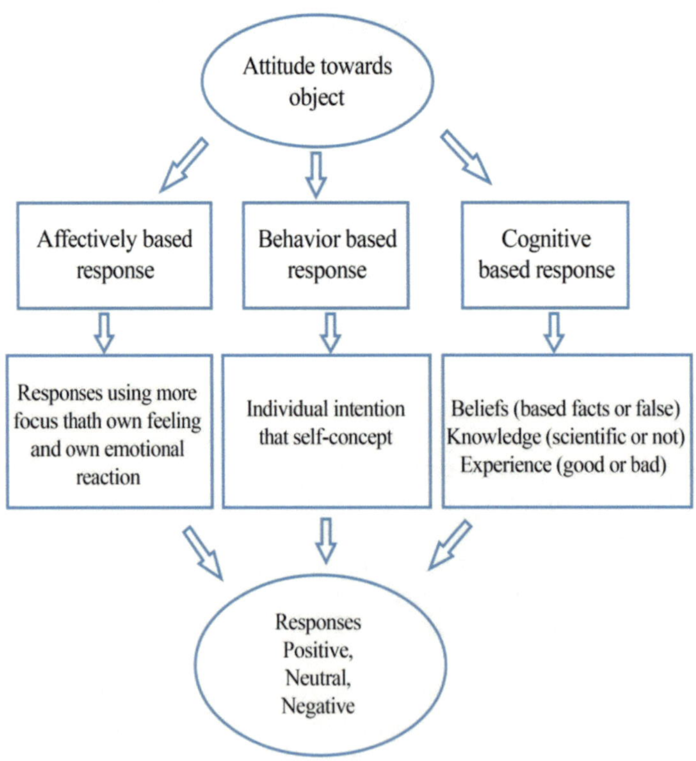

Figure 1.
Response of attitude model by Gelegjamts [10].

Attitudes refer to the positive or negative attitude evaluations that people make about any aspect of reality [11]. Attitudes are directly related to the thoughts and beliefs one has towards object of attitude [6] these beliefs and attitudes can also impact the level of palliative education [12].

Cultural factors of attitudes such as race, religion, ethnicity may also have a perspective effect on a patient's suffering and recovery.

The attitude of healthcare professionals towards dying patients may vary based on their cultural structure, religious thought, social environment, family structure the technology used in their unit, communication methods, palliative care training, and previous experience of encountering death [13].

A supportive care attitude has recognized the psychosocial features and problems that make every patient a unique individual and these unique characteristics can greatly influence suffering and need to be considered when planning caring service [14].

2.2 Measurement of attitude towards object

In 1928 Louis Leon Thurston said, "attitude can be measured" [8] and "attitude can be learned" [6]. Humans are not born with attitudes, and they acquire attitudes during their lifestyle and course of socialization [6]. Attitudes measurements have followed the explicit attitude (acquired consciousness) and the implicit attitude (subconsciously) dichotomy, attitude can be examined through direct and indirect measures [15].

The Implicit attitude measures are more valid and reliable. This has important implications are implicit attitude measures (such as self-reports). The implicit measures help account for attitudes that a person may be aware of or want to show [16] and usually rely on an indirect measure of attitude. The implicit attitudes measurement tests, include the implicit association test, evaluative and semantic priming tasks, the Extrinsic Affective Simon Task, Go/No-Go Association Task, and the Affect Misattribution Procedure. The explicit attitude measures are direct measurement and attitude-related acquired knowledge. The explicit measure is lower valid and more reliable than the implicit measure because people are often unwilling to provide responses perceived as socially undesirable and therefore tend to report what they think their attitude should be rather than what they know them to be [17]. Explicit and Implicit attitudes did not correlate: the model of dual attitudes [18].

The following points highlight the top five techniques used to measure the attitude of an individual. The techniques are [19]:

1. Method of Equal Appearing Interval (Developed by L.L. Thurstone and Chave. 1929)

2. Method of Summated Rating (Developed by Likert)

3. Social Distance Scale (Developed by Katz and Allport under the guidance of Gallet and Bogardus.)

4. Cumulative Scaling Method (Developed by Guttman's cumulative scaling method, 1944)

5. The Scale Discriminating Technique. (Developed by Edwards and Kilpartic.)

Method of summated rating

Likert developed this method of summated rating and is famous for constructing several attitude scales to measure attitudes towards various complex issues.

Liker's scale is presented in five categories such, on a 5-point (Strongly Agree, Somewhat Agree, Neutral, Somewhat Disagree, Strongly Disagree) scale, for example, researchers assume that the psychological difference between Strongly Agree to strongly disagree [6].

The total score for each individual subject for all the statements is calculated by summing up each individual response. The use of 'Item Analysis' in the construction of attitude scale is the most important feature of Likert's scale. In this scale, the individual scores are interpreted in terms of the scores obtained by a group of individuals which is commonly done in psychological test construction.

2.3 Measurement of attitudes towards end of life

Many tools have been developed to measure the attitude for health care professionals such as physicians, nurses, and medical students and the tools usually measure with their knowledge, attitude, and practice (KAP).

It is important to have tools that allow us to know the attitudes of health care professionals towards the care of patients who is under Palliative care [9]. Attitudes towards palliative care were defined as feelings, thoughts, attitudes, and comfort level towards care of the patients and their family [5, 20] and most of the available tools are in attitude and competence in dealing with death and dying tools that are Frommel's attitudes towards care of the dying (FATCOD—A for nurses, FATCOD-B for students) scale by 1991 [21]. FATCOD tool has been used with physicians and nurses form different countries and a few countries' reports have been using for psychologists and social workers [5, 9, 13, 22–24]. This tool is specifically designed for evaluating nurses and has an equal number of positively and negatively worded items and responding rate is 5 point on the Liker scale, ranging from 30 to 150. Higher scores reflected more positive attitudes towards the end of life. It is necessary for health care professionals to better understand death, accept, and prepare for it with a mature attitude [25, 26]. Death attitude profile revised (created by Wong, Reker and Gesser in 1994 [27]) tool is reliable and valid assessment instrument used to identify attitudes about care at the end of life among clinicians [9]. DAP-R reliability values were high and the five domains of attitude towards death i.e., fear of death, death avoidance, natural acceptance, approach acceptance, and escape acceptance, respectively [26, 28].

Additionally, many study has used attitude related tools and scales such as the cancer attitudes questionnaire, the attitude assessment questionnaire, the cancer attitude inventory, and attitudes towards pain.

3. Health care professional's attitude about palliative care for cancer patients

3.1 Introduction about supportive and palliative care among cancer patients

Palliative care (PC) is a specialized medical care for people living with a life terminal illness and provides relief from the symptoms and stress [29] including people who have stopped treatment to cure or control their disease [30]. Anyways the goal of PC is to improve quality of life for both the patient and their family members.

PC and SC (supportive care) are appropriate for not only cancer patients but also those with serious illness, regardless of whether or not they are receiving life-limiting therapies and can be delivered in inpatient and outpatient settings appropriate at any age, at any stage and can be provided together with curative treatment [31]. Palliative care incorporates the whole spectrum of care-medical, nursing, psychological, social, cultural, and spiritual [32]. A holistic approach, including these extensive attitudes of care, which is a good medical practice and in palliative care it, is essential [32]. Palliative care, which has historic roots in end-of-life and hospice care, now has established itself as a medical specialty dedicated to helping patients with serious illness live as well as possible for as long as possible [2].

Supportive care (SC) in cancer is defined as "the prevention and management of the adverse effects of cancer and its treatment and includes management of physical and psychological symptoms and side effects across the continuum of the cancer experience from diagnosis through treatment to post-treatment care [33]. Enhancing rehabilitation, secondary cancer prevention, survivorship, and end-of-life are care integral to supportive care [33]. SC is also helping manage the common side effects of cancer treatment, thereby enhancing the quality of life in patients receiving cancer therapy.

Supportive care is a necessary service for those with cancer to meet their physical, emotional, social, psychological, informational, spiritual, and practical needs during the diagnostic, treatment, and follow-up [34, 35], encompassing issues with survivorship, palliative care, and bereavement [35]. The SC of patients with cancer improves patient's quality of life, increases the patient's survival rate and reduces side effects caused by treatment of a disease [1].

Studies have shown that patients and providers have a more favorable impression of the term "supportive care" than "palliative care." As a result of tremendous advances in the treatment of early and advanced stages, more patients live with a diagnosis of cancer for longer periods of time. Despite improvements in cancer care, however, many patients continue to experience side effects from both their disease and treatment [2].

Both "Palliative care" and "Supportive care" can be given at any point during a person's illness to help them feel more comfortable [15].

PC and SC both work together as a team that focuses on quality of life and holistic services to patients and their family members. Abundant data now demonstrate that Palliative and Supportive care is beneficial to patients and their families and should be more incorporated into cancer care. In particular, patients with advanced cancer have to deal with many problems during the progression of the disease such as pain, fatigue, energy depletion, and loss of appetite, along with physical symptoms of cancer itself. In addition, cancer patients have a variety of psychological symptoms such as being suggestive anxiety, depression, and sleep disorders [34].

Anderson who is a Texas University physician found that the term "palliative care" was perceived as more distressing and as reducing hope for patients and families. They preferred the name "supportive care" and stated that they would be more likely to refer patients to a service named "supportive care" [21]. After the institution changed the name of both inpatient and outpatient services from "palliative care" to "supportive care" in 2007, they found a 41% increase in consults.

In addition, registration of outpatient palliative care services decreased from 13.2 months to 9.2 months, indicating that patients were being seen earlier in the disease process [36]. Researchers from the University of Pittsburgh interviewed patients with advanced cancer and found that patients had a more favorable impression of the term "supportive care" than "palliative care" [37]. The fields of "supportive care" and "palliative care" in oncology emerged from separate patient needs, have since evolved and are now intertwined. Supportive care arose specifically to combat toxicities of cancer treatment [2].

No significant difference was found between specialists who perceived the terms "palliative care" and "supportive care" [38].

3.2 Health care professional's attitudes towards cancer patients

Groot et al., [39] determined three-common barriers to perceiving palliative care services including:

- Barriers relating to knowledge, skills.
- Barriers concerning communication and collaboration teamwork.
- Barriers related to the organization of care.

In Gibbs et al., [40] determined common barriers including lack of adequately trained palliative care physicians, nurses, and social workers; lack of knowledge among patients and families, and lack of training opportunities for existing health-care team members, all of which add to implementation difficulties [41].

Cultural, ethnic, and religious beliefs help to shape people's attitude towards and dying [42]. Cancer patients have physical (physical symptoms), social (social isolation), functional (activity), spiritual (spiritual abandonment), emotional (sadness, anxiety.) wellbeing needs.

Health care professionals (HCP) have to provide positive attitudes towards different needs during an appropriate time for cancer patients. Additionally, cultural values and beliefs play a role in Health care professional's attitudes towards palliative care patients [12, 42, 43].

Mc Loughlin KE studied the healthcare professional's attitudes towards palliative care and caring for dying patients and a number of countries used her studies to measure healthcare professional attitudes including Germany, Denmark, the UK, the Netherlands, Wales, California America [44] and Texas [35].

In 2007 researcher's evidence showed that the attitude of healthcare professionals can change through the provision of palliative care education [45, 46] and through providing palliative care.

A health care professional has a more positive attitude to care for these people which is also associated with less fear and avoidance of death, anxiety, and stress [9, 22–24].

Healthcare professionals have different attitudes towards dying patients, for example, oncologists and nurses had more positive attitudes towards PC and caring for dying patients than other healthcare professionals.

Dr. Kathleen found 5 factors influencing health professionals' attitudes towards palliative care (as shown in **Figure 2**).

Below including

1. Knowledge of palliative care and case to discuss (knowledge)
2. Importance of honesty with patient and recognition of benefits of early referral (communication)

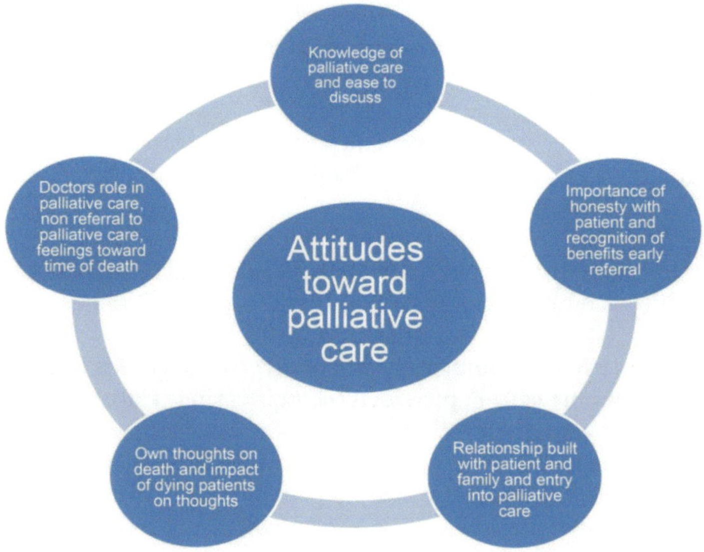

Figure 2.
Factor of attitudes towards palliative care uploaded by Mcloughlin [44].

3. Relationships built with patients and family and entry into palliative care

4. Own thoughts on death and impact of dying patients on thought (culture)

5. Doctor's role in palliative care nonreferral to palliative care feelings towards time of death

They reflect more on existential matters such as nurses being more likely to agree that dealing with a dying patient made them more aware of their own feelings about death than doctors did. In general, nurses were more positive than doctors about palliative care.

In one study of the Danish healthcare professionals, nurses were more likely than doctors to agree that palliative care was a rewarding part of their work and was less likely to prefer to leave the care of dying patients to others [47].

However, most of the studies were assessed the attitude towards dying care and knowledge in palliative care for nurses rather than physicians and health care workers.

There is a need to introduce or reinforce the study of palliative care in the curriculum of medical doctors, nurses, pharmacists, and other healthcare workers both at undergraduate and postgraduate levels.

The improvement of attitudes towards palliative care is crucial to enable healthcare professionals who have a role in referring patients to palliative care, to discuss services in a positive way and facilitate a seamless transition to palliative care as well as reduce fear of death and a sense of failure when referring patients to palliative care [48, 49].

The attitude of professionals has been found to be one of the most significant predictors of quality of care which has a positive impact on quality of life at the end of patients' lives [50]. Negative attitudes create barriers to providing comprehensive patient care [51, 52].

This can cause stress and anxiety for professionals when caring for patients in end-of-life situations, which can affect their own health in the long term [53, 54].

HCP has to know about that:

- The relatives of patients with advanced disease are subject to considerable emotional and physical distress, especially if the patient is being managed at home.

- Particular attention must be paid to their needs as the success or failure of palliative care may depend on the caregiver's ability to cope.

- Palliative care, whether at home or in a hospital, often succeeds or fails to depend on the care and support system provided by their caring relatives.

McLoughlin (2012) identified the attitude towards palliative care highlighted the need to educate the public on issues concerning palliative care. That was consisted with 2014 Nigeria study showing the gaps in the knowledge of healthcare workers in the area of palliative care [30].

3.3 Health care team's attitude towards palliative care

Palliative care is a multi-discipline care system that tries to improve the quality of the patient and relieve them by controlling the symptoms related to the disease [55–57]. Pain and symptom management are the primary focus and psycho-social, spiritual and bereavement support are also provided by multi-discipline teamwork [5]. The basic palliative care teams are made up of physicians and nurses with the support of psychologists and social workers [58]. Additionally include other specialist, nutritionist, pharmacist, chaplain, physiotherapist (as shown in **Figure 3**).

Multi-discipline team provides the patients and their family members with physical, social, and emotional functional support based on the adequate knowledge of PC and favorable attitude towards the end-of-life care.

Positive attitudes towards palliative care are important to enable good communication between primary caregivers and specialist palliative care providers [59].

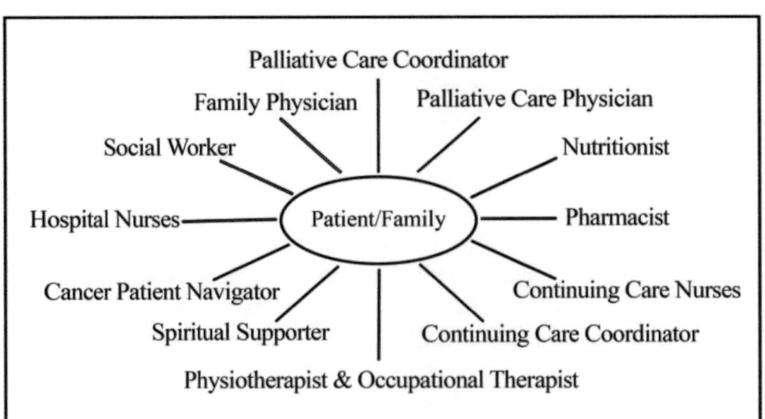

Figure 3.
Ministry of Health USA uploaded by 2011.

In Mongolia, they concluded attitude towards inter-professional education in health care professionals needed more practice training for team efficacy and attitude value [60]. Training in palliative care and previous experience related to the end of life has an influence on improving the attitude of health professionals towards the care of patient's end of life [61].

Health care providers require a good relationship with dying patients and their family members. This is the most difficult process and forming such a relationship is painful as it involves suffering and grieving if the patient passes.

Good communication between all the health care professionals involved in a patient's care is essential and is fundamental to many aspects of palliative care and good communication with patients and families is also essential [32]. Good palliative care helps open up discussion with patients and their families about important aspects of end-of-life care [62]. Healthcare professionals should consider encourage cancer patients of such positive beliefs and though [63].

3.4 Nurses attitude towards palliative care

The palliative care nurses are expected to participant in the multidiscipline team coordinating for patients, but they need structured preparation to feel knowledgeable and comfortable so they can engage in conversations related to palliative care [41]. In 2022 Ethiopian researchers made Conceptual framework on factors associated with nurses' attitude towards nursing profession. Four different factors affecting nurses' attitude towards professional that are socio-demographic factors, organizational related factors, social supporting factors and health professional related factors [64]. Standards of oncology nursing education highlight the need to represent the scope of teaching in all phases of cancer care, including prevention, early detection, rehabilitation, survivorship, and supportive care [41].

Many studies reported a significant correlation between the level of knowledge and attitudes towards palliative care. This is highlighted that as a participants' level of knowledge increased, attitude became more positive either setting in hospitals such as in Lebanon India, Ethiopia, and Saudi Arabia primary care settings such as in Thailand. It is a part of human nature that the degree and complexity of knowledge affect their attitudes and in turn their behavior.

Nurses as well as other health care workers often feel unprepared for their tasks in palliative care and are in much need of more expertise in the field of pain and symptom management, communication, and dealing with ethical dilemmas [65].

Nurses are another key group with widely differing attitudes towards palliative care [55]. Nurses working in older people's care settings such as community hospitals and nursing homes are ideally placed to deliver palliative care [18].

The attitudes of nurses, who are frequently confronted with the phenomenon of death during the day, towards providing services to patients whose death is approaching are important for the quality of the care provided. The attitudes of nurses towards dying patients may vary based on their cultural structure, religious thought, social environment, family structure, the technology used in their unit, communication methods, palliative care training, and previous experience of encountering death [13, 55].

Nurses play an important role in the end-of-life care in attitudes of practices because they are more in direct contact with dying patients and spend more time with patients and their family members than other health care professionals. Additionally, nurse providers nursing problem such as pain, breathing difficulties, nausea, vomiting, and fatigue occurring in when patients need essential clinical care [55].

In1991 Degner et al. [1] determined nursing behavior in care for dying people is responding during the death scene, providing comfort, responding to anger, enhancing personal growth, responding to colleagues, enhancing quality of life during dying, and responding to the family.

3.5 Undergraduate student attitude towards palliative care

Palliative care (PC) education for medical students is very important. Because studies on medical students found that it is stressful dealing with end-of-life patients and coping when discussing bad news and encountering relatives' grief and fear of death. In recent years, medical school faculty have focused on disseminating misconceptions and fears as well as developing positive attitudes towards students' future role in providing PC [66, 67]. Although generally linked to education level and clinical learning, student attitude towards EOL care seem to have a wider range of influences, particularly cultural [68].

Medical students who experienced a patient's death during practice reported significantly more positive attitudes and clinical experience with EOL care was a significant predictor of attitudes in some of the studies taken in Mongolia (2021), Italy (2021), and Indonesia (2020).

Bassah et al. [69] concluded in their review on end-of-life attitudes in nursing students that little time is usually devoted to palliative care education or that it is often included in order specialized nursing courses [9]. The education on end-of-life (EOL) care as a portion of PC is very important for physicians, nurses and health care professionals should be prepared to provide quality EOL care [70]. Furthermore, medical education should prepare future students to meet increased PC about awareness and attitudes needs [71]. Medical education on PC in Asian countries could be improved by students' education from the European Association for Palliative Care or the End-of-Life Nursing Education Consortium.

Moreover, nursing educators could improve their capacity to teach PC courses by attending train-the-trainer sessions and nursing schools could change their curricula to include mandatory PC courses or integrate basic PC education into their curricula. However, teaching strategies may be important in improving the quality of PC education [10].

4. Public attitude towards cancer

4.1 Public impact of attitudes and feelings on cancer

In spite of improving cancer survival rate, decreasing negative attitudes and myths about cancer [72] the thought of impending death [73, 74], social difficulties, and feeling isolated [63] are still around. Cancer survivors need prime support from people close to them to successfully cope with their diagnosis and treatment as well as continual support to improve their quality of life after treatment [75]. Additionally, government and non-government organizations should act to provide a more supportive environment [63, 72], and promote community awareness and intervention activities to enable access to community, social, and individual units for the social reintegration of cancer survivors [76]. In Korean studies from 2012 about public attitudes towards cancer such as cancer stigma, cancer disparities, and stereotypes of cancer. Looking at results of public attitude 58.5% think it is impossible to treat cancer regardless of advanced technology, 71.8% think people with cancer are unable to make contributions to society, and 23.5% of people would avoid working with persons who have cancer [72]. Furthermore in Oman's public study 63% said they faced difficulties in marriage.

In 2007–2011, LIVESTRONG implemented a global cancer research study planned to give people who had a cancer a chance to share their cancer experiences and their view on the cancer problem that is caused by stigma and silence. They analyzed media coverage, public opinion surveys, and semi-structured interviews from Argentina, Brazil, China, France, India, Italy, Japan, Mexico, Russia, and South Africa [77]. Looking at the results, there has to be a positive change for cancer stigma, to improve cancer awareness, promote communication between cancer patients to share cancer experiences, and the education system including cancer awareness such as cancer prevention, early detection, tobacco use, nutrition [77]. Subsidiary also has to have positive change for disparities of cancer and cancer stereotypes [73].

Kathryn conducted a qualitative study on public perception of cancer, a balance of positive and negative beliefs, and concluded that; People appear to be "in two minds" about cancer. A rapid, intuitive sense of dread and imminent death coexist with a deliberative, rational recognition that cancer can be a manageable, or even curable, disease. Recognizing cancer's public image could help in the design of effective cancer control messages [74].

Negative attitudes formed from lifestyle and cultural factors, lack of education, religion, living in rural areas, smokers [75], low monthly income [76], misinformation about cancer screening, lack of health-seeking behaviors [73] and lack of rehabilitation during and after treatment. Patients with a negative attitude about cancer are affected by their quality of life, recovery from cancer, time of treatment, and adequate support from the workplace and society.

Discriminatory behavior towards cancer may isolate patients from their community, complicate returning to work after treatment, and have unfavorable physical and mental health consequences for cancer survivors [73]. Public education should also be focused on myths about cancer, such as the impossibility of recovery, and fear of the disease. In addition, people living with cancer should be encouraged to share their experiences with other people in society [73].

Morse Life Hospice studied people's beliefs and attitudes towards end-of-life care. The top three of awareness included huge support of medical marijuana, opinions on religion, and overall understanding of hospice care. The results show what the public wants and help identifies opportunities to increase awareness in the greater community. The study found that 87% of Americans support the use of medical marijuana as a treatment and believe it is important to have access to a religious leader of their faith for spiritual guidance during their hospice care (72%) [78]. An increasing number of cancer prevention campaigns supported by well-established theories about healthy behaviors have improved public health communication, leading to increased public awareness about the lifestyle risk factors related to cancer.

A positive attitude has also been linked to strong spirituality, religious beliefs, and a keen interest in cancer.

How to improve public role in supporting cancer patients.

(What information do they need to know)

1. Understanding your diagnoses (what is cancer, how cancer is diagnosed, how to advance, how to cope, how do I talk to people about having cancer, etc.)

2. Understanding your Treatment and side effects (preparing for and getting treatment, learning about treatment, dealing with side effects, more information, and resources)

3. Survivorship communication (during and after treatment, cancer survivor course, attending cancer groups, staying active, healthy during and after treatment, and sharing cancer experiences with the same diagnosis person)

4. Learning and forming positive attitudes towards cancer, ignoring feelings such as sadness, distress, depression, fear, and anxiety

5. Conclusions

Attitude is an essential role in palliative care and supportive care for cancer patients. Cancer patients and their family members need a different attitude from other palliative care patients. Especially positive attitude towards cancer patients to improve their quality of life in aspects such as physically, emotionally, spiritually, socially and help them live as long as possible. There are important roles in attitude such as culture, beliefs, and thoughts but attitude can be changed and can be learned by knowledge, and practice. HCP who work within the PC and SC field have to be mentally prepared from when they are students for high knowledge and positive attitude and ability practice.

Author details

Delgersuren Gelegjamts[1,2]* and Batbagana Burenerdene[3]

1 Chosun University, Gwangju, South Korea

2 Medical school of Mongolian National University, Ulaanbaatar, Mongolia

3 Seojeong College, Yanju, South Korea

*Address all correspondence to: degijulie@gmail.com

References

[1] National Cancer Institute. NCI Dictionary of Cancer Terms. Bethesda, Maryland: National Cancer Institute; 2019. Available from: cancer.gov/publications/dictionaries/cancer-terms/def/supportive-care

[2] Shelly S, Lo MD, Mary K, Buss MD. What Is the Difference Between Supportive and Palliative Care? Alexandria, VA: ASCO News; 2019. Available from: https://dailynews.ascopubs.org/do/10.1200/ADN.19.190354/

[3] Gysels M, Evans N, Meñaca A, Andrew E, Toscani F, Finetti S, et al. Culture and end of life care: A scoping exercise in seven European countries. PLoS One. 2012;**7**(4):e34188. DOI: 10.1371/0034188

[4] Fang ML, Sixsmith J, Sinclair S, Horst G. A knowledge synthesis of culturally-and spiritually-sensitive end-of-life care: Findings from a scoping review. BMC Geriatrics. 2016;**16**(1):1-4. DOI: 10.1186/s12877-016-0282-6

[5] Kim JS, Kim J, Gelegjamts D. Knowledge, attitude and self-efficacy towards palliative care among nurses in Mongolia: A cross-sectional descriptive study. PLoS One. 2020;**15**(7):e0236390. DOI: 10.1371/0236390

[6] Perloff RM. The Dynamics of Persuasion: Communication and Attitudes in the Twenty-First Century. 6nd ed. Oxfordshire, United Kingdom: Taylor & Francis; 2016. DOI: 10.4324/9781315657714

[7] Perloff RM. The Dynamics of Persuasion: Communication and Attitudes in the Twenty-First Century. 7th ed. Oxfordshire, United Kingdom: Taylor & Francis; 2020. DOI: 10.4324/9780429196959

[8] Wight RD, Gable PA. Encyclopedia of Statistics in Behavioral Science. Vol. 4. London: Wiley; 2005. pp. 2045-2046

[9] Herrero-Hahn R, Román-Calderón JP, Montoya-Juárez R, Pérez-Cuervo P, García-Caro MP. Frommelt attitude toward care of the dying scale form B: Validation for Spanish health professionals. Palliative and Supportive Care. 2021:1-9. DOI: 10.1017/S1478951521001504

[10] Gelegjamts D, Yong Yoo J, Kim J, Sun KJ. Undergraduate nursing students' palliative care knowledge and attitudes towards end-of-life care: A cross-sectional descriptive study. Contemporary Nurse. 2020;**56**(5-6):477-490. DOI: 10.1080/10376178.2021.1890165

[11] Brinol P, Petty RE, Valle C, Rucker DD, Becerra A. The effects of message recipients' power before and after persuasion: A self-validation analysis. Journal of Personality and Social Psychology. 2007;**93**(6):1040. DOI: 10.1037/0022-3514.93.6.1040

[12] Wang L, Li C, Zhang Q, Li Y. Clinical nurses' attitudes towards death and caring for dying patients in China. International Journal of Palliative Nursing. 2018;**24**(1):33-39. DOI: 10.12968/ijpn.2018.24.1.33

[13] Eues SK. End-of-life care: Improving quality of life at the end of life. Professional Case Management. 2007;**12**(6):339-344. DOI: 10.1097/01.0000300408.00325.1c

[14] IAHPC. Guiedelines and Suggesting for those Starting a Hospice Palliative

Care Service. Houston, TX, USA: IAHPC; 2021. Available from: https://hospicecare.com/what-we-do/publications/getting-started/SBN - 978-0-9989787-5-8

[15] Available from: https://en.wikipedia.org/wiki/Attitude

[16] Kassa H, Murugan R, Zewdu F, Hailu M, Woldeyohannes D. Assessment of knowledge, attitude and practice and associated factors towards palliative care among nurses working in selected hospitals, Addis Ababa, Ethiopia. BMC Palliative Care. 2014;**13**(1):6. DOI: 10.1186/1472-684X-13-6

[17] Das A, Haseena T. Knowledge and attitude of staff nurses regarding palliative care. International Journal of Science and Research (IJSR). 2015;**4**(11):1790-1795

[18] Wilson RS, Bennett DA, Bienias JL, Aggarwal NT, Mendes De Leon CF, Morris MC, et al. Cognitive activity and incident AD in a population-based sample of older persons. Neurology. 2002;**59**(12):1910-1914. DOI: 10.1212/01.0000036905.59156

[19] Measuring the Attitude of an Individual: Top 5 Techniques. 2021. Available from: https://www.psychologydiscussion.net/attitudes/measuring-the-attitude-of-an-individual-top-5-techniques/1362

[20] Frommelt KHM. The effects of death education on nurses' attitudes toward caring for terminally ill persons and their families. American Journal of Hospice & Palliative Medicine. 1991;**8**(5):37-43. DOI: 10.1177/ 104990919100800509

[21] Fadul N, Elsayem A, Palmer JL, Del Fabbro E, Swint K, Li Z, et al. Supportive versus palliative care: what's in a name? A survey of medical oncologists and midlevel providers at a comprehensive cancer center. Cancer. 2009;**115**(9): 2013-2021. DOI: 10.1002/24206

[22] Espinoza-Venegas M, Luengo-Machuca L, Sanhueza-Alvarado O. Attitudes held by Chilean nursing professionals on care of the dying. A multivariate analysis. Aquichan. 2016;**16**(4):430-446. DOI: 10.5294/2016.16.4.3

[23] Bermejo JC, Villacieros M, Hassoun H. Attitudes towards end of life patient care and fear of death in a healthcare student sample. Spain: Medicina Paliativa; 2018. DOI: 10.1016/2017.02.004

[24] Barnett MD, Reed CM, Adams CM. Death attitudes, palliative care self-efficacy, and attitudes toward care of the dying among hospice nurses. Journal of Clinical Psychology in Medical Settings. 2020:1-6. DOI: 10.1007/s10880-020-09714-8

[25] Kim YH, Ahn SY, Lee CH, et al. Development of a death education curriculum model for the general public using dacum method. Technology and Health Care. 2016;**24**(3):439-446

[26] Xu F, Huang K, Wang Y, Xu Y, Ma L, Cao Y. A questionnaire study on the attitude towards death of the Nursing interns in eight teaching hospitals in Jiangsu, China. BioMed Research International. 2019;**2019**:3107692

[27] Wong PT, Reker GT, Gesser G. Death attitude profile-revised: A multidimensional measure of attitudes toward death. Death Anxiety Handbook: Research, Instrumentation, and Application. 1994;**121**:121-148

[28] Brudek P, Sekowski M, Steuden S. Polish adaptation of the death attitude profile-revised. Omega (Westport)-Journal of Death and Dying. 2018;**81**(1):18-36

[29] About Palliative Care. 2020. Available from: https://www.capc.org/about/palliative-care/

[30] Blaževičienė A, Laurs L, Newland JA. Attitudes of registered nurses about the end-of- life care in multi-profile hospitals: a cross sectional survey. BMC Palliative Care. 2020;**19**(1):131. DOI: 10.1186/s12904-020-00637-7

[31] Available from: https://getpalliativecare.org/whatisPalliativecareon,providedalongwithcurativetreatment

[32] Available from: https://hospicecare.com/what-we-do/publications/getting-started/principles-of-palliative-care/

[33] Multinational Association of Supportive Care in Cancer. What is MASCC? . Available from: www.mascc.org/about-mascc [Accessed February 29, 2016]

[34] Park SA, Chung SH, Shin EH. Attitudes of nurses toward supportive care for advanced cancer patients. Asian Pacific Journal of Cancer Prevention. 2012;**13**(10):4953-4958. Available from: http://journal.waocp.org/article_26973

[35] Hui D. Definition of supportive care: Does the semantic matter? Current Opinion in Oncology. 2014;**26**(4):372-379. DOI: 10.1097/CCO.0000000000000086

[36] Dalal S, Palla S, Hui D, Nguyen L, Chacko R, Li Z, et al. Association between a name change from palliative to supportive care and the timing of patient referrals at a comprehensive cancer center. The Oncologist. 2011;**16**(1):105-111. DOI: 10.1634/theoncologist.2010-0161

[37] Maciasz RM, Arnold RM, Chu E, Park SY, White DB, Vater LB, et al. Does it matter what you call it? A randomized trial of language used to describe palliative care services. Supportive Care in Cancer. 2013;**21**(12):3411-3419. DOI: 10.1007/s00520-013-1919-z

[38] Hui D, Park M, Liu D, Reddy A, Dalal S, Bruera E. Attitudes and beliefs toward supportive and palliative care referral among hematologic and solid tumor oncology specialists. The Oncologist. 2015;**20**(11):1326-1332. DOI: 10.1634/theoncologist.2015-0240

[39] Groot MM, Vernooij-Dassen MJ, Crul BJ, Grol RP. General practitioners (GPs) and palliative care: Perceived tasks and barriers in daily practice. Palliative Medicine. Mar 2005;**19**(2):111-118

[40] Gibbs Jr KD, Mahon MM, Truss M, Eyring K. An assessment of hospital-based palliative care in Maryland: Infrastructure, barriers, and opportunities. Journal of Pain and Symptom Management. 1 Jun 2015;**49**(6):1102-1108

[41] Harden K, Price D, Duffy E, Galunas L, Rodgers C. Palliative care: Improving nursing knowledge, attitudes, and behaviors. Clinical Journal of Oncology Nursing. 2017;**21**(5):E232-E238. DOI: 10.1188/17.CJON.E232-E238

[42] Jafari M, Rafiei H, Nassehi A, Soleimani F, Arab M, Noormohammadi MR. Caring for dying patients: Attitude of nursing students and effects of education. Indian Journal of Palliative Care. 2015;**21**:192-197. DOI: 10.4103/0973-1075.156497

[43] Koppel M, Onwuteaka-Philipsen BD, van der Steen JT, Kylanen M, Van den Block L, Smets T, et al. Care staff's self-efficacy regarding end-of-life communication in the long-term care setting: Results of the PACE

cross-sectional study in six European countries. International Journal of Nursing Studies. 2019;**92**:135-143. DOI: 10.1016/j.ijnurstu.2018.09.019

[44] McLoughlin KE. Identifying and Changing Attitudes toward Palliative Care: An Exploratory Study (Doctoral Dissertation). Maynooth, Ireland: National University of Ireland Maynooth; 2012

[45] Frommelt KH. Attitudes toward care of the terminally ill: an educational intervention. American Journal of Hospice and Palliative Medicine®. 2003;**20**(1):13-22

[46] Wessel EM, Rutledge DN. Home care and hospice nurses' attitudes toward death and caring for the dying: Effects of palliative care education. Journal of Hospice & Palliative Nursing. 2005;7(4):212-218

[47] Vejlgaard T, Addington-Hall JM. Attitudes of Danish doctors and nurses to palliative and terminal care. Palliative Medicine. 2005;**19**(2):119-127

[48] Raudonis BM. Palliative care update for gastroenterology nurses. Gastroenterology Nursing. 2003;**26**(1):26-30. DOI: 10.1097/00001610-200301000-00006

[49] Hanratty B, Hibbert D, Mair F, May C, Ward C, Corcoran G, et al. Doctors' understanding of palliative care. Palliative Medicine. 2006;**20**(5):493-497. DOI: 10.1191/0269216306pm1162oa

[50] Ascencio EJ, Cieza-Gómez GD, Carrillo-Larco RM, Ortiz PJ. Timed up and go test predicts mortality in older adults in Peru: A population-based cohort study. BMC Geriatrics. 2022;**22**(1):61. DOI: 10.1186/s12877-022-02749-6

[51] Ascencio-Lane JC, Smart D, Lippmann J. A 20-year analysis of compressed gas diving-related deaths in Tasmania, Australia. Diving and Hyperbaric Medicine. 2019;**49**(1):21-29. DOI: 10.28920/dhm49.1.21-29

[52] Sadowska M, Sarecka-Hujar B, Kopyta I. Cerebral palsy: Current opinions on definition, epidemiology, risk factors, classification and treatment options. Neuropsychiatric Disease and Treatment. 2020;**16**:1505-1518. DOI: 10.2147/NDT.S235165

[53] Caton AP, Klemm P. Introduction of novice oncology nurses to end-of-life care. Clinical Journal of Oncology Nursing. 2006;**10**(5):604-608. DOI: 10.1188/06.CJON.604-608

[54] Shoji K, Cieslak R, Smoktunowicz E, Rogala A, Benight CC, Luszczynska A. Associations between job burnout and self-efficacy: A meta-analysis. Anxiety, Stress, and Coping. 2016;**29**(4):367-386. DOI: 10.1080/10615806.2015.1058369

[55] Akbolat M, Ünal Ö, Karakaya BG. Turkish adaptation of the Frommelt attitude toward care of the dying scale. OMEGA—Journal of Death and Dying. 2020;**84**(4):1160-1174

[56] Kabalak AA, Öztürk H, Çağıl H. Yaşam sonu bakım organizasyonu; palyatif bakım. Yoğun Bakım Dergisi. 2013;**11**(2):56-70

[57] Finkel M. Ellerby K. No Shortcut to Change: An Unlikely Path to a More Gender-Equitable World. New York, NY: New York University Press; 2017. 288 pp., $30 (paperback). ISBN: 9781479817160. Journal of Women, Politics & Policy. 2018;39(3):396-8.

[58] Ministry of Health. Palliative Care Strategy of the National Health System. 2011. 2010-2014 Update. Available from:

http://www.msps.es/organizacion/sns/planCalidadSNS/docs/paliativos/cuidadospaliativos.pdf

[59] Shipman C, Burt J, Ream E, Beynon T, Richardson A, Addington-Hall J. Improving district nurses' confidence and knowledge in the principles and practice of palliative care. Journal of Advanced Nursing. Sep 2008;**63**(5):494-505

[60] Baatar A, Nyamjav S, Sandag O. Attitudes toward interprofessional education and collaborative practices in Mongolia. International Journal on Integrated Education. 2020;**3**(8):48-52

[61] Dimoula M, Kotronoulas G, Katsaragakis S, Christou M, Sgourou S, Patiraki E. Undergraduate nursing students' knowledge about palliative care and attitudes towards end-of-life care: A three-cohort, cross-sectional survey. Nurse Education Today. 2019;**74**:7-14. DOI: 10.1016/j.nedt.2018.11.025

[62] Kim Y, Yoo SH, Shin JM, Han HS, Hong J, Kim HJ, et al. Practical considerations in providing end-of-life care for dying patients and their family in the era of COVID-19. American Journal of Hospice & Palliative Medicine (AJHPM). 2021;**24**:130-134. DOI: 10.14475/jhpc.2021.24.2.130

[63] Al-Azri M, Al-Hattali F, Al-Ghafri H, Panchatcharam SM. Attitudes towards cancer patients: A cross-sectional study of Omani patients and attendees at a university teaching hospital. Sultan Qaboos University Medical Journal. 2021 May;**21**(2):e221-e230. DOI: 10.18295/squmj.2021.21.02.010

[64] Rekisso AD, Mengistu Z, Wurjine TH. Nurses' attitudes towards the nursing profession and associated factors in selected public hospitals, Addis Ababa, Ethiopia, 2021: A cross-sectional study. BMC Nursing. 2022;**21**:21. DOI: 10.1186/s12912-022-00808-2

[65] Armes PJ, Addington-Hall JM. Perspectives on symptom control in patients receiving community palliative care. Palliative Medicine. 2003;**17**(7):608-615. DOI: 10.1191/0269216303pm801oa

[66] Gibbins J, McCoubrie R, Maher J, Wee B, Forbes Recognizing K. That it is part and parcel of what they do: Teaching palliative care to medical students in the UK. Palliative Medicine. 2010;**24**:299-305

[67] Barclay S, Whyte R, Thiemann P, Benson J, Wood DF, Parker RA, et al. An important but stressful part of their future work: Medical Students' attitudes to palliative care throughout their course. Journal of Pain and Symptom Management. 2015;**49**(2):231-242

[68] Max E, Mackenzie M. Just in KASE: Evaluating nursing students' knowledge, attitudes and self-efficacy to care for the dying patient (S721). Journal of Pain and Symptom Management. 2017;**53**(2):421

[69] Bassah N, Seymour J, Cox K. A modified systematic review of research evidence about education for pre-registration nurses in palliative care. BMC Palliative Care. 2014;**13**(1):56. DOI: 10.1186/1472-684X-13-56

[70] American Association of Colleges of Nursing. Competencies and Recommendations for Educating Undergraduate Nursing Students (CARES): Preparing Nurses to Care for the Seriously Ill and their Families. Washington, D.C., United States: AACN; 2016

[71] Ferrell B, Malloy P, Mazanec P, Virani R. CARES: AACN's new competencies and recommendations for educating undergraduate nursing students to improve palliative care.

Journal of Professional Nursing. 2016;**32**(5):327-333. DOI: 10.1016/j.profnurs.2016.07.002

[72] Cho J, Smith K, Choi EK, Kim IR, Chang YJ, Park HY, et al. Public attitudes toward cancer and cancer patients: A national survey in Korea. Psycho-Oncology. 2013;**22**(3):605-613. DOI: 10.1002/pon.3041

[73] Badihian S, Choi EK, Kim IR, Parnia A, Manouchehri N, Badihian N, et al. Attitudes toward cancer and cancer patients in an urban Iranian population. The Oncologist. 2017;**22**(8):944-950

[74] Robb KA, Simon AE, Miles A, et al. Public perceptions of cancer: A qualitative study of the balance of positive and negative beliefs. BMJ Open. 2014;**4**:e005434. DOI: 10.1136/bmjopen-2014005434

[75] Kye SY, Lee HJ, Lee Y, Kim YA. Public attitudes towards cancer survivors among Korean adults. Cancer Research and Treatment: Official Journal of Korean Cancer Association. 2020;**52**(3):722

[76] Shim HY, Shin JY, Kim JH, Kim SY, Yang HK, Park JH. Negative public attitudes towards cancer survivors returning to work: A nationwide survey in Korea. Cancer Research and Treatment. 2016 Apr;**48**(2):815-824. DOI: 10.4143/crt.2015.094

[77] Livestrong Report. Cancer Stigma and Silence Around the World. 2011. Available from: http://www.livestrong.org/pdfs/3-0/LSGlobalResearchReport [Accessed: May 2014]

[78] Available from: https://morselife.org/morselife-hospice-and-palliative-care-survey-findings-reveal-attitudes-about-medical-marijuana-religion-and-end-of-life-care/

Chapter 6

Perspective Chapter: Palliative Surgery in Pediatric Cancer

Alessandro Inserra and Cristina Martucci

Abstract

Childhood can cer survival rates have lately improved (from 54% in 1980 to an actual 80%), and palliative care has taken on a larger role in the management of oncological kids, with many clinicians involved (including oncologists, radiologists, and surgeons). Palliative surgery has evolved from "noncurative" treatments to a variety of surgeries used to relieve organ dysfunction and provide the best possible quality of life in all aspects of life (clinical, psychological, and social).

Keywords: palliative, surgery, children, cancer

1. Introduction

Palliative surgical oncology, which is widely developed in adult care, is a new issue in children, whose treatment should include not only the patients but also their relatives.

Palliative care is defined by the World Health Organization (WHO) as "an approach that improves the quality of life of patients and their families facing the problem of life-threatening illness through the prevention and relief of suffering through early identification and impeccable assessment and treatment of pain and other physical, psychosocial, and spiritual problems" [1]. This statement emphasizes the need of treating oncological children comprehensively.

2. The application of palliative care in pediatric patients

The word "palliative" comes from the Latin terms "pallium" (which represents the dress or overcoat of ancient Roma) and "palliation" (which means "to cloak or cover"); in medicine, the concept of cloaking or covering has been employed not to "hide" but to "protect" the person, in a vision of protective care [2].

Pediatric oncology represents a huge success in the story of medicine, with an overall survival rate of 80%. Recently, many progress has been made in pediatric palliative protocols, incorporating multidisciplinary support in physical, emotional, spiritual, mental, social, and financial aspects, highlighting the significance of comprehensive palliative care teams and management programs [3, 4]. Recent medical advances in South Africa have demonstrated that effective multidisciplinary palliative care involving children's families and communities can be implemented successfully even in resource-limited settings, usually through voluntary and unstructured forms of activities and participations [5–7].

The Wayne State University School of Medicine established the first hospital-based palliative care consult service in the United States in 1985 at Detroit Receiving Hospital; Dr. Declan Walsh established the first palliative medicine program in the United States in 1987 at the Cleveland Clinic Cleveland, Ohio: it was the first wide-ranging integrated program designated as a WHO international demonstration project and accredited by the European Society of Medical Oncology. Following it, several other programs were established, including the Palliative Care Program at the Medical College of Wisconsin (1993), the Pain and Palliative Care Service at Memorial Sloan-Kettering Cancer Center (1996), and The Lilian and Benjamin Hertzberg Palliative Care Institute at Mount Sinai School of Medicine (1997). Since then, there has been a considerable increase in the number of hospital-based palliative care programs, which now number over 1400. Currently, 80% of US hospitals with more than 300 beds have a palliative care program [8].

Palliative care was not available for children for many decades, and only a few pediatric patients have recently benefited from a dedicated palliative care service [3, 9]. It can be used in a variety of fields, including:

- Clinical: monitoring of symptoms and signs, balancing relief of adverse events with avoidance of unnecessary hospitalizations without compromising the quality of life;

- Psychological: patient and family support, clear communication, dealing with emotional issues (understanding, acceptance, anger, self-confidence, etc). The care plan should encourage personality development, the preservation of daily routines, the achievement of targets, and the setting of realistic future goals;

- Social: providing opportunities for entertainment, allowing the child to remain an active school participant and an age-appropriate socially functional community member, and promoting spiritual and religious fulfillment.

The role of surgery in palliative care is to achieve the best quality of life for cancer patients for as long as possible; surgeons may participate in oncological management in a variety of ways, including obtaining correct and representative biopsies to confirm histological diagnosis, positioning central venous catheters for short- or long-term use and nutritional devices, and performing curative or tumor-debulking surgeries (reducing symptoms caused by tumor compression on adjacent structures) [10]. Furthermore, based on clinical aspects and tumor peculiarities, each patient must have a unique, tailored management plan. "How far is too far?", "What is far enough?", and "How far is not far enough?" are among the numerous questions that remain for surgical management of palliative care patients. Ethical conflict is vital, especially when choosing on tumor debulking and removal of malignant metastases in palliative patients: each decision must be founded on the child's and family's values and rights, as well as the beliefs, duties, and rights of all parties involved [11].

Moreover, Kassam A. et al. found that adolescents and young adults with cancer (particularly hematological disorders) have a greater rate of intensive care at the end-of-life stage than adults in a recent publication (40.6% vs. 22.4%) [12]. Oncological kids die in hospitals over half of the time (and nearly half of them in intensive care units), compared to only 25% of adults who die in hospitals. Furthermore, pediatric patients dying of oncological disease usually suffer greatly in their final weeks of life: according to parental reports, 89% of these children have at least one debilitating symptom, particularly weariness, discomfort, or dyspnea, till the end of their lives [13, 14].

These findings may reflect professionals' discomfort and lack of experience with advanced care planning discussions, deferred conversations about end-of-life (in order to protect younger patients), and caregiver pressure to continue treatments (even if they are ineffective) at the end of their child's life [15, 16]. It may be challenging for the surgeon to pick the appropriate care for their patients in this highly emotional and demanding scenario.

The American College of Surgeons [17] issued a statement on the values of palliative care in August 2005, which was based on the following principles:

1. Respect the dignity and autonomy of patients, patients' surrogates, and caregivers;

2. Honor the right of the competent patient or surrogate to choose among treatments, including those that may or may not prolong life;

3. Communicate effectively and empathically with patients, their families, and caregivers;

4. Identify the primary goals of care from the patient's perspective and address how the surgeon's care can achieve the patient's objectives;

5. Strive to alleviate pain and other burdensome physical and nonphysical symptoms;

6. Recognize, assess, discuss, and offer access to services for psychological, social, and spiritual issues;

7. Provide access to therapeutic support, encompassing the spectrum from life-prolonging treatments through hospice care, when they can realistically be expected to improve the quality of life as perceived by the patient;

8. Recognize the physician's responsibility to discourage treatments that are unlikely to achieve the patient's goals and encourage patients and families to consider hospice care when the prognosis for survival is likely to be less than half a year;

9. Arrange for continuity of care by the patient's primary and/or specialist physician, alleviating the sense of abandonment patients may feel when "curative" therapies are no longer useful;

10. Maintain a collegial and supportive attitude toward others entrusted with care of the patient.

Pain, bleeding, intestinal or urinary obstruction, malnutrition, lack of vascular access, fluid collections, intracranial hypertension, respiratory distress, infections, and selective intra-tumoral therapies are just a few of the conditions that may necessitate surgical intervention in oncological patients.

2.1 Pain

Pain is one of the most pressing concerns for children with cancer, as it has a significant impact on their quality of life [18]. It is one of the most concerning and widespread symptoms, with prevalence rates ranging from 24–60% of patients during chemotherapy and 62–86% in advanced-stage cancer, indicating that the problem has yet to be solved [13, 19]. Furthermore, according to a recent meta-analysis, more than one-third of patients with pain describe it as moderate to severe (VAS >4), and while many authors distinguish between cancers with a high risk of pain (bone, pancreas, and esophagus) and cancers with a low risk of pain (lymphoma, leukemia, and soft tissue), no significant correlation has been found between pain prevalence and cancer type. There were no changes in the prevalence of pain between senior and younger patients [20].

Aside from physical concerns, a variety of variables might influence how you feel. Pain management is important in palliative care because cancer pain is multifactorial and can present with a variety of other symptoms. It should include pharmacological, medical, biopsychosocial, and even surgical approaches (such as debulking procedures to reduce tumoral compression/stimulation of nerves or ganglions). To study each clinical case and establish a customized "pain-relieving" strategy, a multidisciplinary surgical team (e.g. surgeons, anesthesiologists, radiologist, interventionist, and nursing staff) is required [21].

WHO developed a "Three-Step Analgesic Ladder" to demonstrate proper analgesic use in adult patients [22], with three levels:

1. Simple analgesics (acetaminophen [paracetamol] and nonsteroidal anti-inflammatory drugs);

2. Minor opioids (codeine and tramadol);

3. Major opioids (morphine, diamorphine, and fentanyl).

In pediatrics, however, it is recommended to use analgesics in two steps, depending on the degree of the pain: paracetamol and ibuprofen should be used first for children with light pain; in patients with moderate to severe pain, an opioid may be considered [23].

Analgesics from the following step up should be added or substituted as the pain intensity increases and the current analgesics are no longer sufficient. Adjuvant therapies, such as anticonvulsant medication for neuropathic pain, should be added at all stages.

The authors of a recent multicenter study based in the United Kingdom found that patients dying of solid tumors are more likely to receive high doses of opioids; this circumstance could be related to the biology of these neoplasms, which can compress nerves or metastasize to bone in the late stages, causing pain: in fact, pain was more common in children with solid tumors (98.4%) than in others (87%) [24].

Other instruments that can aid in the pain management of cancer patients include:

- *Intrathecal therapy*: individuals with refractory cancer pain or unbearable side effects may benefit from intrathecal morphine sulfate delivery via an implanted patient-activated delivery system [25–27];

- *Epidural analgesic administration*: As previously documented by many authors (such as Plancarte R. in 1991 and Portas M. in 1998) [28, 29], epidural opioid injection should be investigated in children with intractable body pain to minimize discomfort and improve long-term analgesia [30–32];

- *Peripheral nerve block*: neurolytic plexus blockage (i.e. celiac or brachial plexus) may be conducted on children with malignancies whose pain is inadequately controlled with oral medications or who have uncontrollable adverse effects (such as opiod toxicity), as stated by several authors [33]. According to Chambers W.A [34], about 8–10% of patients may benefit from a peripheral nerve block, and about 2% from a central neuraxial block; additionally, some patients may benefit from a simple peripheral block relieving just one component of their pain [33].

- *Cryoablation and radiofrequency*: these procedures are routinely investigated for malignant painful lesions in the axial/appendicular skeleton and in a variety of soft tissue. They are less commonly employed in pediatric palliative care [35]. According to Ferrer-Mileo L.et al. systematic's review [36], they may reduce mean pain scores and the demand for opioids, therefore enhancing the quality of life.

- *Cordotomy*: Cordotomy was first described in 1912, and it was performed by interrupting the spinothalamic route many layers above the painful location with an open surgical procedure. This procedure, which has now evolved into a minimally invasive percutaneous image-guided needle cordotomy, is an effective and selective surgical treatment for intractable cancer pain; it consists in inserting a needle in the upper cervical spinal cord at the C1–C2 level under CT guidance in order to reach the antero-lateral quadrant of the opposite side. Electrical stimulation is used to check for coverage of painful body locations and current-induced paresthesias. Percutaneous cordotomy complications, such as hemiparesis and dysesthesia, have become extremely rare, and mortality is nearly nonexistent. However, no reports of application in the pediatric population have been made, most likely due to the need for active participation in the process to ensure proper needle positioning during intraoperative stimulation [37–39].

- *Neuromodulation procedures*: recentlyvarious stimulating devices have been developed, even if it is yet unknown the exact mechanism producing the antalgic impact of electrical stimulation: possibilities include activation of GABAergic neurons and recruitment of multimodality transmitting sensory pathways [40]. Anesthesiologists can readily place these devices percutaneously in the epidural space, and they can be used at various levels of the neurological system. Electrodes for peripheral nerves are also available, but they usually necessitate an open surgical operation. Because stimulation intensity and frequency are modifiable factors, all of these methods have the advantage of reversibility and personalization of treatment. Infection risk, high expenses, and the invasiveness of surgical procedures are all major drawbacks [41].

- *Midline myelotomy*: this procedure could be used as a substitute for a cordotomy, which can be done openly (via a laminotomy) or by a percutaneous needle method. Interrupting the crossing of spinothalamic fibers in the midline allows for the control of bilateral pain, making it the usual method for both bilateral and visceral pain [37].

Despite all of the various therapies to oncological pain, a number of studies have found that 40–70% of patients had insufficient pain control [42, 43]. The Agency for Health Care Policy and Research's "First Barriers National Clinical Practice Guidelines on Cancer Pain" [44] clearly describes and categorizes the barriers to proper cancer pain treatment into three groups:

a. System barriers: Low priority given to cancer pain treatment, legal and regulatory barriers to the use of opioids for cancer pain (due to concerns about opioid abuse and addiction) [45], insufficient or late start of palliative care program, high cost of opioids, and challenges with treatment availability or access.

b. Professional barriers: Failure to follow guidelines and lack of medical education, analgesia level based on prognosis rather than pain severity, fear of patient addiction and analgesic tolerance, lack of proactive questioning about the symptom, insufficient experience with pain management.

c. Patient barriers: Reluctance to disclose pain, recognition of increased levels of pain suggesting disease progression, fear of being labeled as "bad patient," fear of addiction, tolerance, and opioid adverse effects.

Based on WHO standards, two metrics for evaluating analgesic adequacy have been created:

- Morphine Consumption Data: because morphine is the medicine of choice for the management of severe cancer pain, it is a common indication of how well cancer pain is handled on a national and worldwide basis [46];

- Pain Management Index (PMI) [47]: when the patient's reported level of pain and the necessary prescribed analgesics are in agreement, pain management is termed adequate. The patient describes the pain using a numerical rating scale from 0 to 10 and the symptom is then classified into four categories:

1. No pain;

2. Mild pain [1–4];

3. Moderate pain [5–6];

4. Severe pain [7–10].

The analgesic drug prescribed is similarly classified at one of four levels:

1. No analgesics;

2. Non-opioid analgesics;

3. Weak opioids

4. Strong opioids.

The PMI is calculated by subtracting the pain level from the analgesic level. Scores will range from −3 to 3: negative scores are an indicator of undertreatment, while a score of 0 is considered acceptable as a minimal level of treatment.

2.2 Bleeding

Bleeding can be a life-threatening complication in pediatric oncology patients, necessitating rapid blood transfusions and/or definitive hemorrhage control (by surgery, embolization, or devascularization) [48]. Bleeding was recorded in 12.7% of the investigated population (particularly in hematological patients) in the UK Children's Cancer Study Group/Pediatric Oncology Nurses Forum Survey of 2006 [49], but only a handful of them required surgical operations. Selective arterial embolization (SAE) may be a safer and more successful method of treating acute hemorrhages in children with cancer than surgery, which can be too intrusive and carry a high risk of morbidity and mortality in patients with severe illnesses [50].

2.3 Bowel obstruction

In oncological children, bowel blockage normally progresses over time, although it can also be abrupt. Symptoms are connected to irregular intestinal transit (abdominal distension, bilious/fecaloid vomiting, and dehydration) and can quickly affect the patient's clinical state and the quality of life [51]. Bowel obstruction can be caused by a variety of factors, including tumor growth compressing the gut, intra-luminally blocking masses, radiotherapy side effects, past surgery complications, or harsh medical treatment creating intestinal stenosis or occlusion. The goal of treatment should be to relieve abdominal distention, clear the blockage (restore bowel continuity and/or bypass the "obstacle"), and avoid consequences (dyselectrolytemia, bacterial overgrowth, and perforation) as well as respiratory distress (caused by increase of intra-abdominal pressure) [52]. Even while an intestinal stoma can be a source of additional trauma for oncological children and their parents, it can also help to improve the quality of life by providing a viable option for nutritional needs (through gastrostomy), bolus or continuous enteral feedings. Although most patients tolerate bolus feeding, intolerance can manifest itself in the form of vomiting, severe abdominal distension, excessive gastric residuals, or diarrhea. If this is the case, continual feedings are required, especially in patients who are at high risk of aspiration or have poor absorption [53].

2.4 Urinary obstruction

Urinary obstruction occurs in nearly 10% of adults with advanced primary or metastatic intra-abdominal cancer, according to recent literature; no data on this issue has been documented in the pediatric population. Pelvic neuroblastoma, vesical or prostatic rhabdomyosarcoma, abdominal Burkitt lymphoma, non-Hodgkin lymphoma, retroperitoneal germ cell tumors, diffuse desmoplastic tumor, and peritoneal metastatic disease are the most common cancers that can cause urinary obstruction in children. Furthermore, periureteral fibrosis, a long-term side effect of chemo and radiation therapy, may exacerbate the situation. Urinary blockage can be influenced by a variety of factors, including: tumor development caused by recurrent, metachronous, or metastatic disease; tumor blockage caused by extraluminal carcinomatosis or bulk; tumor intramural growth; tumor direct adhesion or kinking. Urinary blockage symptoms include abdominal pain, oliguria/anuria, ascites increasing hydronephrosis, and a high serum creatinine level. It denotes a situation that necessitates immediate urine relief or diversion (depending on the degree of obstruction) using:

Open urinary diversion: Surgical alternatives include laparotomy for tumor debulking and/or urinary tract resection with anastomosis or stoma and suprapubic cystostomy for individuals with a favorable prognosis, good performance level, and a single site of obstruction.

Retrograde ureteral stent: In individuals with a short life expectancy, a percutaneous nephrostomy tube, such as an internal double J nephro-ureteric stent (double J) or an internal/external nephroureteral stent (NUS), is advised [54].

Nephrostomy tube: In patients who are not candidates for surgery, a percutaneous nephrostomy should considered.

There are currently few data on the true occurrence of this complication in intra-abdominal malignancies, resulting in a lack of therapy guidelines [55, 56]. Even in these circumstances, a multidisciplinary team of specialists is needed, including pediatric surgeons, urologists, radiologists, interventionists, and medical oncologists.

2.5 Malnutrition

Malnutrition is an unfavorable side effect of cancer treatment. Weight loss happens in 41.3% of children with cancer, and nutritional supplementation is required in some cases. In many circumstances, nutritional needs are met by administering total parenteral nutrition (TPN) through central venous catheters; in other cases, enteral feeding via a nasogastric/orogastric tube or gastrostomy/jejunostomy is an option [57, 58].

2.6 Vascular access

Vascular access is a major concern in the treatment of children with cancer [59–62]. Vascular access can be divided into two categories:

- Peripheral: intravenous fluids, medicine, blood product delivery, and blood collection are all indications for peripheral vascular lines.

- Central: TPN, chemotherapy, long-term medication, emergency access, critical care monitoring, dialysis, and extracorporeal membrane oxygenation are all done with them (ECMO). The involvement of the surgeon in their insertion is critical, but so is flawless management by competent experts.

2.7 Fluid collections

Persistent ascites is uncommon in children and is usually caused by past surgery or congenital lymphatic system problems. To minimize abdominal distension, diaphragm raising, and respiratory difficulty, refractory ascites may necessitate surgical interventions. Fluid accumulation in other organ systems (chest, heart, liver, etc.) can lead to organ dysfunction, failure, and, in the worst-case scenario, multi-organ failure.

When medical treatments (bed rest, diet changes, drugs, and fluid restriction) fail, surgical options include fluid drainage or shunting (paracentesis, pleurocentesis, cardiocentesis, chest drains, perito-venous shunt, transjugular intrahepatic portosystemic shunt—TIPS), and even organ transplantation [63]. Every procedure must be incorporated in a wider vision of palliative care, balancing between the best therapy and the quality of life of the kid.

While ultrasound-guided paracentesis is normally reserved for patients who are toward the end of their lives [64], cuffed tunneled peritoneal catheters can be used for long-term external drainage in patients who have a longer life expectancy. A peritoneal catheter joined to a subcutaneous port or completely implanted perito-neovenous (PVS) shunting (such as the Denver shunt) may be used as an alternate instrument for intermittent aspiration in rare cases [65].

Malignant pleural effusion is also a major issue in cancer children's palliative care. The most common treatments for treating oncological children with life-threatening pleural effusions are repeated thoracentesis, pleurodesis, or insertion of pleural drainage [66, 67].

2.8 Intracranial hypertension

Solid organ tumors account for around 30% of all malignancies in children, with brain tumors being the most frequent. Intracranial hypertension is the most aggressive indicator of central nervous system (CNS) neoplasms, and it can produce neurological symptoms such as seizures, worsening levels of awareness, and debilitation [68]. Shunting (ventriculo-peritoneal or ventriculo-atrial shunting) to reduce intracranial pressure can improve the quality of life, and drainage to reduce pressure (EVD-external ventricular drain) can be performed if shunting is contraindicated. These surgical operations must be proposed with caution, taking into account all parties involved in the child's palliative care plan. Each surgical intervention in a successful palliative care plan should strike a balance between proper pain and symptom control and avoiding unnecessary extension of suffering [69].

2.9 Respiratory complications

Almost 11% of advanced tumors in children cause upper respiratory tract compression [70]; in these circumstances, a tracheostomy should be performed to alleviate child discomfort, allow more effective airway suctioning and simpler movement, and simplify the capacity to speak and feed orally. Caregivers and patients should always be included in the surgical planning process to ensure the best stoma management and an acceptable quality of life, free of prejudice, and prejudice [71, 72].

2.10 Infections

Infections should be managed using the same principles as palliative care for children with cancer. Infections must be treated aggressively in order to eliminate the cause of infection (e.g. debridement, abscess drainage, and wound care). Blood cultures are required if central line-associated bloodstream infections (CLABSI) are suspected, and if confirmed, a decision on whether to remove, replace, or leave the line in place should be made [73].

2.11 Selective intra-tumoral/intra-lesional therapies

The surgical team in the palliative care program for children with cancer should not overlook this issue. The intra-arteriolar chemo-infusion by super-selective catheterization of the involved area in retinoblastoma is a well-known example [74];

transcatheter selective arterial chemoembolization (TACE) as adjuvant preoperative treatment for unresectable or chemoresistant hepatoblastoma is another one [75].

3. Conclusion

The following are the main principles of surgical palliative care in pediatric cancer patients:

- Respect the patient's life, health, and autonomy;
- Maximize the benefit to the patient while minimizing the harm;
- Always act professionally, fairly, rationally, and honestly;
- Each patient must have a tailored care plan that adheres to the principles discussed.

Success in surgical palliative care for oncological children includes assisting the child and their families in living as well as possible and then, at the end of life, helping the patient in dying quietly.

"Death isn't a medical failure, it's a biological certainty. But poorly managed death IS a medical failure." (Dr. Kathryn Mannix).

Author details

Alessandro Inserra and Cristina Martucci*
Ospedale Pediatrico Bambino Gesù, IRCCS, Rome, Italy

*Address all correspondence to: cristina.martucci@opbg.net

References

[1] Sepulveda C, Marlin A, Yoshida T, Ullrich A. Palliative care: The World Health Organization's global perspective. Journal of Pain and Symptom Management. 2002;**24**(2):91-96

[2] Saga Y, Enokido M, Iwata Y, Ogawa A. Transitions in palliative care: Conceptual diversification and the integration of palliative care into standard oncology care. Chinese Clinical Oncology. 2018;**7**(3):32

[3] Feudtner C, Kang TI, Hexem KR, et al. Pediatric palliative care patients: A prospective multicenter cohort study. Pediatrics. 2011;**127**(6):1094-1101

[4] Back A, Friedman T, Abrahm J. Palliative care skills and new resources for oncology practices: Meeting the palliative care needs of patients with cancer and their families. American Society of Clinical Oncology Educational Book. 2020;**40**:1-9

[5] Radbruch L, De Lima L, Knaul F, et al. Redefining palliative care-a new consensus-based definition. Journal of Pain and Symptom Management. 2020;**60**(4):754-764

[6] Wearne N, Davidson B, Motsohi T, Mc Culloch M, Krause R. Radically rethinking renal supportive and palliative care in South Africa. Kidney International Reports. 2020;**6**(3):568-573

[7] Amery JM, Rose CJ, Holmes J, Nguyen J, Byarugaba C. The beginnings of children's palliative care in Africa: Evaluation of a children's palliative care service in africa. Journal of Palliative Medicine. 2009;**12**(11):1015-1021

[8] Roth AR, Canedo AR. Introduction to hospice and palliative care. Primary Care. 2019;**46**(3):287-302

[9] Laronne A, Granek L, Wiener L, Feder-Bubis P, Golan H. Oncologist conceptualizations of pediatric palliative care: Challenges and definitions. Supportive Care in Cancer. 2021;**29**(7):3981-3989

[10] Inserra A, Narciso A, Paolantonio G, Messina R, Crocoli A. Palliative care and pediatric surgical oncology. Seminars in Pediatric Surgery. 2016;**25**(5):323-332

[11] Inserra A, Crocoli A. Palliative care: A surgicalperspective. Pediatric Blood & Cancer. 2019;**66**(8):e27817

[12] Kassam A, Gupta A, Rapoport A, et al. Impact of palliative care involvement on end-of-life care patterns among adolescents and young adults with cancer: A population-based cohort study. Journal of Clinical Oncology. 2021;**39**(22):2506-2515

[13] Daut RL, Cleeland CS. The prevalence and severity of pain in cancer. Cancer. 1982;**50**(9):1913-1918

[14] Wolfe J, Grier HE, Klar N, et al. Symptoms and suffering at the end of life in children with cancer. The New England Journal of Medicine. 2000;**342**(5):326-333

[15] MacKenzie AR, Lasota M. Bringing life to death: The need for honest, compassionate, and effective end-of-life conversations. American Society of Clinical Oncology Educational Book. 2020;**40**:1-9

[16] Long KA, Patterson P, Fainsilber Katz L, Amaro CM, Alderfer MA. Creating a pathway for psychosocial support in siblings of youth with a chronic illness: Findings from an international summit. Journal of Developmental and Behavioral Pediatrics. 2021;**42**(4):331-339

[17] Dunn GP. Surgery, palliative care, and the american college of surgeons. Annals of Palliative Medicine. 2015;**4**(1):5-9

[18] Miser AW, Dothage JA, Wesley RA, Miser JS. The prevalence of pain in a pediatric and young adult cancer population. Pain. 1987;**29**(1):73-83

[19] van den Beuken-van Everdingen MH, de Rijke JM, Kessels AG, Schouten HC, van Kleef M, Patijn J. Prevalence of pain in patients with cancer: A systematic review of the past 40 years. Annals of Oncology. 2007;**18**(9):1437-1449

[20] van den Beuken-van Everdingen MH, Hochstenbach LM, Joosten EA, Tjan-Heijnen VC, Janssen DJ. Update on prevalence of pain in patients with cancer: Systematic review and meta-analysis. Journal of Pain and Symptom Management. 2016;**51**(6):1070-1090.e9

[21] Neufeld NJ, Elnahal SM, Alvarez RH. Cancer pain: A review of epidemiology, clinical quality and value impact. Future Oncology. 2017;**13**(9):833-841

[22] Reid C, Davies A. The World Health Organization three-step analgesic ladder comes of age. Palliative Medicine. 2004;**18**(3):175-176

[23] Tutelman PR, Chambers CT, Stinson JN, et al. Pain in children with cancer: Prevalence, characteristics, and parent management. The Clinical Journal of Pain. 2018;**34**(3):198-206

[24] Goldman A, Hewitt M, Collins GS, Childs M, Hain R. United Kingdom Children's Cancer study group/paediatric oncology Nurses' forum palliative care working group. Symptoms in children/young people with progressive malignant disease: United Kingdom children's cancer study group/paediatric oncology nurses forum survey. Pediatrics. 2006;**117**(6):e1179-e1186

[25] Rauck RL, Cherry D, Boyer MF, Kosek P, Dunn J, Alo K. Long-term intrathecal opioid therapy with a patient-activated, implanted delivery system for the treatment of refractory cancer pain. The Journal of Pain. 2003;**4**(8):441-447

[26] Coyne PJ, Smith T, Laird J, Hansen LA, Drake D. Effectively starting and titrating intrathecal analgesic therapy in patients with refractory cancer pain. Clinical Journal of Oncology Nursing. 2005;**9**(5):581-583

[27] Deer TR, Levy R, Prager J, et al. Polyanalgesic consensus conference--2012: Recommendations to reduce morbidity and mortality in intrathecal drug delivery in the treatment of chronic pain. Neuromodulation. 2012;**15**(5):467-482

[28] Portas M, Marty JY, Buttin C, et al. Refractory pain in children with cancer: Role of peridural analgesia. Archives de Pédiatrie. 1998;**5**(8):851-860

[29] Plancarte R, Patt R. Intractable upper body pain in a pediatric patient relieved with cervical epidural opioid administration. Journal of Pain and Symptom Management. 1991;**6**(2):98-99

[30] Tsui BC, Berde CB. Caudal analgesia and anesthesia techniques in children. Current Opinion in Anaesthesiology. 2005;**18**(3):283-288

[31] Aram L, Krane EJ, Kozloski LJ, Yaster M. Tunneled epidural catheters for prolonged analgesia in pediatric patients. Anesthesia and Analgesia. 2001;**92**(6):1432-1438

[32] Baker L, Lee M, Regnard C, Crack L, Callin S. Tyneside spinals group. Evolving spinal analgesia practice in palliative care. Palliative Medicine. 2004;**18**(6):507-515

[33] Cooper MG, Keneally JP, Kinchington D. Continuous brachial

plexus neural blockade in a child with intractable cancer pain. Journal of Pain and Symptom Management. 1994;**9**(4):277-281

[34] Chambers WA. Nerve blocks in palliative care. British Journal of Anaesthesia. 2008;**101**(1):95-100

[35] Lessard AM, Gilchrist J, Schaefer L, Dupuy DE. Palliation of recurrent Ewing sarcoma of the pelvis with cryoablation and somatosensory-evoked potentials. Journal of Pediatric Hematology/ Oncology. 2009;**31**(1):18-21

[36] Ferrer-Mileo L, Luque Blanco AI, Gonzalez-Barboteo J. Efficacy of cryoablation to control cancer pain: A systematic review. Pain Practice. 2018;**18**(8):1083-1098

[37] Mullan S, Harper PV, Hekmatpanah J, Torres H, Dobbin G. Percutaneous interruption of spinal-pain tracts by means of a Strontium90 needle. Journal of Neurosurgery. 1963;**20**:931-939

[38] Kanpolat Y, Ugur HC, Ayten M, Elhan AH. Computed tomography-guided percutaneous cordotomy for intractable pain in malignancy. Neurosurgery 2009;64(3 Suppl):ons187-ons193

[39] Raslan AM, Cetas JS, McCartney S, Burchiel KJ. Destructive procedures for control of cancer pain: The case for cordotomy. Journal of Neurosurgery. 2011;**114**(1):155-170

[40] Tasker RR. Identification of pain processing systems by electrical stimulation of the brain. Human Neurobiology. 1982;**1**(4):261-272

[41] Meyerson BA, Linderoth B. Mechanisms of spinal cord stimulation in neuropathic pain. Neurological Research. 2000;**22**(3):285-292

[42] Foley KM. How well is cancer pain treated? Palliative Medicine. 2011;**25**(5):398-401

[43] van den Beuken-van Everdingen MH, de Rijke JM, Kessels AG, Schouten HC, van Kleef M, Patijn J. Prevalence of pain in patients with cancer: A systematic review of the past 40 years. Annals of Oncology. 2007;**18**(9):1437-1449

[44] Management of cancer pain: Adults. Agency for health care policy and research. Clinical Practice Guideline. Quick Reference Guide for Clinicians. 1994;**9**(9):1-29

[45] Maltoni M. Opioids, pain, and fear. Annals of Oncology. 2008;**19**(1):5-7

[46] Hewitt M, Goldman A, Collins GS, Childs M, Hain R. Opioid use in palliative care of children and young people with cancer. The Journal of Pediatrics. 2008;**152**(1):39-44

[47] Thronaes M, Balstad TR, Brunelli C, et al. Pain management index (PMI)- does it reflect cancer patients' wish for focus on pain? Supportive Care in Cancer. 2020;**28**(4):1675-1684

[48] Johnstone C, Rich SE. Bleeding in cancer patients and its treatment: A review. Annals of Palliative Medicine. 2018;**7**(2):265-273

[49] Goldman A, Hewitt M, Collins GS, Childs M, Hain R. United Kingdom Children's Cancer study group/paediatric oncology Nurses' forum palliative care working group. Symptoms in children/ young people with progressive malignant disease: United Kingdom children's cancer study group/paediatric oncology nurses forum survey. Pediatrics. 2006;**117**(6):e1179-e1186

[50] ZeghalSouki D, Touhami O, Rajhi H, et al. Selective arterial embolization

in case of bleeding in advanced cervical cancer. La Tunisie Médicale. 2013;**91**(8-9):558-559

[51] Badgwell BD, Contreras C, Askew R, Krouse R, Feig B, Cormier JN. Radiographic and clinical factors associated with improved outcomes in advanced cancer patients with bowel obstruction. Journal of Palliative Medicine. 2011;**14**(9):990-996

[52] Davis M, Hui D, Davies A, et al. Medical management of malignant bowel obstruction in patients with advanced cancer: 2021 MASCC guideline update. Supportive Care in Cancer. 2021;**29**(12):8089-8096

[53] Cousins SE, Tempest E, Feuer DJ. Surgery for the resolution of symptoms in malignant bowel obstruction in advanced gynaecological and gastrointestinal cancer. Cochrane Database of Systematic Reviews. 2016;**2016**(1):CD002764

[54] Allen DJ, Longhorn SE, Philp T, Smith RD, Choong S. Percutaneous urinary drainage and ureteric stenting in malignant disease. Clinical Oncology. 2010;**22**(9):733-739

[55] Sountoulides P, Mykoniatis I, Dimasis N. Palliative management of malignant upper urinary tract obstruction. Hippokratia. 2014;**18**(4):292-297

[56] Geisler JP, Perry RW, Ayres GM, Holland TF, Melton ME, Geisler HE. Ovarian cancer causing upper and lower urinary tract obstruction. European Journal of Gynaecological Oncology. 1994;**15**(5):343-344

[57] Hebuterne X, Lemarie E, Michallet M, de Montreuil CB, Schneider SM, Goldwasser F. Prevalence of malnutrition and current use of nutrition support in patients with cancer. JPEN Journal of Parenteral and Enteral Nutrition. 2014;**38**(2):196-204

[58] Arends J, Baracos V, Bertz H, et al. ESPEN expert group recommendations for action against cancer-related malnutrition. Clinical Nutrition. 2017;**36**(5):1187-1196

[59] Crocoli A, Martucci C, Persano G, et al. Vascular access in pediatric oncology and hematology: State of the art. Children. 2022;**9**(1):70

[60] Crocoli A, Cesaro S, Cellini M, et al. In defense of the use of peripherally inserted central catheters in pediatric patients. The Journal of Vascular Access. 2021;**22**(3):333-336

[61] Crocoli A, Martucci C, Sidro L, et al. Safety and effectiveness of subcutaneously anchored securement for tunneled central catheters in oncological pediatric patients: A retrospective study. The Journal of Vascular Access. 2021;(6):11297298211009364. DOI: 10.1177/11297298211009364 [Online ahead of print]

[62] Crocoli A, Tornesello A, Pittiruti M, et al. Central venous access devices in pediatric malignancies: A position paper of italian association of pediatric hematology and oncology. The Journal of Vascular Access. 2015;**16**(2):130-136

[63] Becker G, Galandi D, Blum HE. Malignant ascites: Systematic review and guideline for treatment. European Journal of Cancer. 2006;**42**(5):589-597

[64] Hodge C, Badgwell BD. Palliation of malignant ascites. Journal of Surgical Oncology. 2019;**120**(1):67-73

[65] Tamagawa H, Aoyama T, Inoue H, et al. Therapeutic results of Denver percutaneous peritoneovenous shunt in cancer patients with malignant ascites.

Journal of Cancer Research and Therapeutics. 2020;**16**(Supplement): S95-S98

[66] Skok K, Hladnik G, Grm A, Crnjac A. Malignant pleural effusion and its current management: A review. Medicina. 2019;**55**(8):490

[67] Ferreiro L, Suarez-Antelo J, Alvarez-Dobano JM, Toubes ME, Riveiro V, Valdes L. Malignant pleural effusion: Diagnosis and management. Canadian Respiratory Journal. 2020;**2020**:2950751

[68] Shimony N, Martinez-Sosa M, Osburn B, Jallo GI. Non-traumatic pediatric intracranial hypertension: Key points for different etiologies, diagnosis, and treatment. Acta Neurologica Belgica. 2021;**121**(4):823-836

[69] Fernandez-Garcia MA, Cantarin-Extremera V, Andion-Catalan M, et al. Secondary intracranial hypertension in pediatric patients with leukemia. Pediatric Neurology. 2017;**77**:48-53

[70] Rowbottom L, Chan S, Zhang L, et al. Impact of dyspnea on advanced cancer patients referred to a palliative radiotherapy clinic. Supportive Care in Cancer. 2017;**25**(9):2691-2696

[71] Abdelaal Ahmed Mahmoud M Alkhatip A, Younis M, Jamshidi N, et al. Timing of tracheostomy in pediatric patients: A systematic review and meta-analysis. Critical Care Medicine. 2020;**48**(2):233-240

[72] Sagiv D, Nachalon Y, Mansour J, et al. Awake tracheostomy: Indications, complications and outcome. World Journal of Surgery. 2018;**42**(9):2792-2799

[73] Rosati P, Saulle R, Amato L, et al. Mindful organizing as a healthcare strategy to decrease catheter-associated infections in neonatal and pediatric intensive care units. A systematic review and grading recommendations (GRADE) system. The Journal of Vascular Access. 2021;**22**(6):955-968

[74] Shields CL, Kaliki S, Rojanaporn D, Al-Dahmash S, Bianciotto CG, Shields JA. Intravenous and intra-arterial chemotherapy for retinoblastoma: What have we learned? Current Opinion in Ophthalmology. 2012;**23**(3):202-209

[75] Li JP, Chu JP, Yang JY, Chen W, Wang Y, Huang YH. Preoperative transcatheter selective arterial chemoembolization in treatment of unresectable hepatoblastoma in infants and children. Cardiovascular and Interventional Radiology. 2008;**31**(6): 1117-1123

Chapter 7

Ethics in Palliative Care

Metin Dincer

Abstract

Health services received at the end-of-life (EoL) are accepted as a basic human right. EoL is a very difficult period for patients and their families. Patients in the EoL period should be provided palliative care (PC) services that will increase their quality of life, so their families. Especially pain and other symptoms that the patient faces should be relieved during PC, and grief counseling should be provided to families in the mourning period after the patient's death. A significant majority of patients who need PC services are cancer patients. Health professionals, including doctors in the first place, should conduct their relationships between patients' families and with patients who need PC in accordance with biomedical ethical principles. The biomedical ethical principles that will protect the boundaries that should not be exceeded are as follows: (1) explaining that the person can participate in decisions about their treatment: Respect for autonomy; (2) explaining that they should not suffer any healthcare-related harm while receiving healthcare services: Nonmaleficence; (3) explaining that the health services they receive should be evidence-based and useful for the patient: Beneficence; and (4) explaining that the patient can get the health service she needs as much as she needs: Justice.

Keywords: end-of-life, palliative care, biomedical ethics, autonomy, nonmaleficence, beneficence, justice

1. Introduction

At the present time, relieving the pain and suffering of terminally ill patients is a basic human right [1]. However, accessing this right is unfortunately not given equal importance all around the world. In a world where death is inevitable, people deserve to die with dignity, that is, to die a "good death." This includes making their own choices, not prolonging death unnecessarily, being considered a complete individual, and giving importance to their family and values [2].

Palliative care (PC) centers have become increasingly important as places that strive to provide a decent death. Their numbers have increased over time since they first emerged, but they are still not at the desired level [3].

Societies have taken their share of the advances in science and technology, which has affected the demographic structure, increased the elderly population and changed the disease patterns. Starting from developed countries, communicable diseases have left their place to non-communicable diseases [4]. These new balances have led to a higher number of healthcare professions and healthcare professionals, and this has made healthcare services more and more complex [5]. Aside from all these, society's expectations of modern medicine have changed, particularly in developed western countries, deaths at home have been replaced with deaths at hospitals [6], which has required ever more careful consideration of the relationship between patients and healthcare professionals.

Morality refers to a set of local norms, rules, and values that are developed by societies to regulate human relations. Ethics, on the other hand, universally refers to a philosophical reflection or questioning about morality, and it is divided into two categories: theoretical ethics and applied ethics [7].

2. Palliative care

Although the history of PC services dates back many years, the first hospice in modern times was opened in the United Kingdom in 1967, and then it spread first to Western Europe and then to the rest of the world [8, 9]. The modern PC has emerged thanks to the groundbreaking work of Dame Cicely Saunders and the Hospice Movement that she started [10].

PC centers provide end-of-life services. This end of life is also referred to as terminal illness, with no common definition or clear time frame for when it occurs [11]. The National Cancer Institute defines the end of life as [12] "care given to people who are near the end of life and who no longer receive treatment to cure or control their disease."

56.8 million people worldwide need PC services, more than half of whom have priority [3]. Twenty-eight percent to 38% of these individuals are cancer patients [3, 13]. For terminally ill cancer patients who receive PC services, the last 6 months of their lives are particularly important, as their physical condition worsens and their symptoms get heavier, and during this time, their physicians tend to explain their prognosis [14–17].

The definition of PC is significant for presenting a framework for the service to be provided. This definition has evolved over time, taking its present form. Though defined by other authors before, the first definition was published by the WHO in 1990 [18], followed by a PC definition for children in 1998 [19]. By 2002, the definitions of PC for adults and children were revised [20] and in 2020, the current definition of PC has become as follows [3]:

> *"Palliative care is an approach that improves the quality of life of patients (adults and children) and their families who are facing the problems associated with life-threatening illness, through the prevention and relief of suffering by means of early identification and correct assessment and treatment of pain and other problems, whether physical, psychosocial or spiritual."*

It includes a comprehensive healthcare delivery system that involves preventive, curative, and rehabilitative health promotion services and PC services [5]. Hence, PC should be considered a healthcare need and a part of comprehensive healthcare services [21, 22]. Based on the definition, some characteristics of PC services include the following. Associated with life-threatening diseases, PC services pay more attention to the social aspect of patients compared to other healthcare services. Besides, the aim is to eliminate the patient's complaints and to increase their quality of life in their final days, rather than treatment. While doing this, PC considers the physical, psychosocial, and spiritual wishes of the patient. A higher quality of life for the patient will increase the quality of life of their loved ones. For example, the patient and their loved ones will be able to go out and have a meal together or spend time in a park in nice weather. While other healthcare services center around the patient and their treatment, PC also considers the patient's close circle, their family, and the grieving process of the family.

Some other characteristics are not included in the definition of PC [3]: it considers death a normal process; it does not try to accelerate or delay death, rather it involves supporting the family in mourning after the patient's death.

Patients' relatives may have different expectations from PC. For example, some might expect PC services to prolong the patient's life rather than improve their quality of life. This does not fit the original philosophy of PC and causes numerous ethical problems, which will be mentioned further in this article.

3. Biomedical ethical principles

Tom L. Beauchamp and James F. Childress have defined four basic biomedical ethical principles [23]: (1) Respect for autonomy; (2) Nonmaleficence; (3) Beneficence; and (4) Justice.

3.1 Respect for autonomy

Autonomy (self-governance, self-rule) is a person's ability to manage themselves and to express their opinion freely regarding decisions about them, without being subject to external pressure [24]. Autonomy also involves the knowledge one has about the medical procedures that will be applied to them. Here, the source of information is the physicians, and the receiver is the patients. However, there is an asymmetry of information between patients and physicians, which occurs when one party has more information about the transaction than the other one, which may allow the better-informed party to use the less-informed party [25].

Information asymmetry is a situation where patients have far less knowledge than physicians, who specialize in the subjects of diseases, treatment options, expected outcomes, and even costs [26]. In this context, autonomy includes the individual's abilities, skills, and characteristics that involve self-management capacities like understanding, reasoning, and negotiating the information given to them about the medical procedures to be performed, and being able to manage and make independent choices about these procedures [23]. Therefore, the principle of respect for patients' autonomy means that each patient has the right to determine which medical interventions they accept or refuse, in other words, decide on the things that affect their own lives [27].

This medical decision-making capacity has four key elements [28]: (1) understanding the benefits, risks, and alternatives of a proposed treatment or intervention, (2) being able to evaluate what these benefits, risks, and alternatives entail, (3) being able to reason and make decisions, and (4) being able to express their choices. If a patient is to undergo a treatment or intervention, or if they are to receive no treatment, their medical decision-making capacity should be considered [28, 29].

With advanced age and diseases like cancer and dementia, cognitive functions tend to suffer, which creates serious obstacles to autonomy [30, 31]. This becomes more evident towards the end of life and largely requires the appointment of a proxy to make decisions on behalf of the patient [32].

The principle of respect for autonomy emerges in an application, which is called "informed consent," in medical ethics, with two aspects (two ways): one of these aspects is informing the patient to eliminate the information asymmetry, and the other is informing patients and obtaining their "consent" about the relevant treatments or interventions [7].

In the process of informed consent, insufficient information is the most important threat to the rationality of patients' medical decisions. This presents as an inability to explain or understand the information. In the first stage of informed consent, the patient must fully comprehend the information given to him/her by the physicians. Medical expressions and medical facts often have a distinct jargon, and they need to be simplified. This simplification may not always be appropriate for the patient, resulting in messages not being fully answered. In the second stage, other conditions like the patient's education level, knowledge level, the severity of their illness or pain, and their level of consciousness can make it difficult to understand what is told.

3.2 Nonmaleficence

Based on the former principle, a new one has emerged. Often attributed to Hippocrates, "primum non nocere" (above all, [first] do no harm) constitutes the basic principle of this new discipline regarding patient safety [33, 34]. "Patient safety is not only state of the art but also a new standard of care" [35]. "Patient safety is freedom from accidental injury" [36] or "patient safety is the prevention of harm to patients" [35]. Based on these definitions, nonmaleficence practices are those that prevent accidental or preventable injuries that might be caused by medical services that are performed to improve patients. Here, the harm done to the patient may result in nothing, or it may result in death.

The "To Err Is Human" report published by the Institute of Medicine in 2000 reported medical error as the eighth most common cause of death for 44,000–98,000 people, which was a complete shock [36]. This report was significant for expressing this fact so clearly for the first time. Another research observed that medical errors were the third most common cause of death with 251,000 deaths [37].

The principle of nonmaleficence involves not only the damage to the individual directly by healthcare services but also the damage that can emerge in various layers of the society due to the misuse of resources, in other words, negative externality. For example, having limited cancer screening programs due to a lack of resources will create a lower incidence of early diagnosis of cancer. Some of these cases will be diagnosed in the advanced stage of the disease, which will require extra time, effort, and costs for treatment. Another example is antibiotic resistance, which increases due to excessive and unnecessary antibiotic use in clinics, requiring newer and more expensive antibiotics.

3.3 Beneficence

The utilitarian ethical theory emphasizes the justification of maximizing people's well-being [38]. Ethics requires that we not only respect people's autonomy and avoid harming them but also contribute to their well-being [23]. Given that improving the quality of life for the patient and their family is the focal point of PC services, this has a crucial perspective. Beneficence is a moral duty to do the best for patients' welfare and to put their well-being first [39].

To be able to fully implement the principle of beneficence, decisions must be based on evidence, because such decisions are much more likely to be fairer. Practicing evidence-based medicine means integrating individual clinical expertise with a critical evaluation of the most relevant external clinical evidence from systematic research [40]. In medicine, the most common ethical dilemmas are about what constitutes patient well-being and who should decide it, which often lead to the concept of respect for patient autonomy [27].

3.4 Justice

According to the Organization for Economic Co-operation and Development, healthcare expenditures continue to increase every year [41], and the unlimited needs of humans are tried to be met with scarce resources, which have caused significant problems. How these resources are allocated to healthcare providers and then prioritized for specific services and patients are some critical ethical decisions that determine the type of healthcare a society receives [42]. In this context, the principle of justice is considered "distributive justice," which refers to the fair, equitable, and appropriate distribution of the benefits and burdens determined by the norms that structure the conditions of social cooperation [23].

The WHO defines justice in healthcare as follows: "the absence of unfair, avoidable, or remediable differences in health status among population groups defined socially, economically, demographically, or geographically" [43]. Here, the concept of justice deems it necessary for those involved to be able to benefit from healthcare services as much as they need without preventing equality of access to healthcare services [44].

Another key issue for resource use is deciding where and how the resources should be allocated. Here, the following questions should be answered [42]: (1) Which healthcare service will be produced for whom and how much? (2) By whom, how, and where will these services be produced? (3) How will society undertake the financial burden of these services? and (4) How will the power and regulation of these services be distributed? In medicine, this means equal distribution of resources to all layers and individuals of the society, both for the healthcare policies that include the whole society, like public health and for therapeutic institutions [7].

4. Other medical ethical principles

Aside from the four basic biomedical ethical principles, we will discuss the following ethical principles: medical confidentiality, truth-telling, and futility.

4.1 Medical confidentiality

In a trust-based patient-physician relationship, medical confidentiality is a fundamental prerequisite that goes back to the Hippocratic oath [45]. Putting forth that physicians must keep their patients' secrets, the principle of medical confidentiality is one of the most respected moral obligations in medical ethics [46]. Medical confidentiality involves respecting the privacy of others regarding their health and keeping their secrets; those who do not fulfill this obligation face criminal sanctions in many countries. A physician-patient relationship is primarily characterized by medical confidentiality, which means that physicians must remain silent about their patients' information [47].

4.2 Truth-telling

The patient-physician relationship and communication are based on trust and telling the truth is a key way to develop and maintain this trust [48]. Telling the truth is often considered a virtue and there is almost a universal phenomenon that physicians are obliged to tell the truth and not lie [49]. Kant assumes that it is a prominent duty, to tell the truth, and deontologically, competent patients must be told the truth, no matter the consequences [50]. The obligation, to tell the truth, is accompanied by a sign of respect for the patient's autonomy. For such cases, the question is how patients can learn the truth about themselves, given that they are entitled to full and accurate information about their medical condition [51]. For example, after diagnosing a life-threatening illness, it may seem appealing and sensible to tell the patient that it can be cured by other physicians, avoiding delivering bad news by eliminating or minimizing the severity of the condition, but it is absolutely unacceptable from an ethical perspective [52]. Still, hiding information from patients, deliberately giving false information, lying, and delivering false information without lying have occurred in nursing and medical practices for centuries [53, 54].

4.3 Futility

Most oncology patients can receive various supportive treatments to have their lives extended for a short time, which brings along prolonged suffering [55]. When treatment becomes meaningless, such treatment decisions should be reviewed. Withdrawal or withholding of life-sustaining treatment decisions are common across emergency departments and adult, pediatric, and neonatal intensive care units, and they are often made before most deaths occur [56]. Withdrawal or withholding of life-sustaining treatment cannot be considered murder or suicide [57], nor passive euthanasia [55].

Withdrawal or withholding of life-sustaining treatment has been increasingly used in institutions that provide end-of-life care [58]. Conceptually, withholding refers to the discontinuation of a treatment that is deemed necessary for living, while withdrawal refers to the discontinuation of a life-sustaining treatment [59]. Though both concepts are used together in this context, withdrawal seems more appropriate at the end of life [60]. In the intensive care units in North America and Europe, life-sustaining treatment has some form of limitation, but end-of-life practices are highly variable [61].

The futility approach is not a new concept; its discussion in the medical and ethical literature began in the 1980s [62]. "Physicians have been advised by Hippocrates to *refuse to treat those who are overmastered by their disease, realizing that in such cases medicine is powerless*" [63, 64]. According to Lo et al., physicians are advised to limit treatment for these four reasons: "the treatment is futile, the patient declines the treatment, the quality of life is unacceptable, or the costs are too great" [62]. According to Trotter, for medical futility to occur, three conditions must be met: setting a target, undertaking an action to achieve this target, and determining the certainty that the action will fail [65].

There is no mutually agreed definition for medical futility, as most definitions tackle the concept from different perspectives. One definition goes as follows:

"a physician's prognostic pronouncement that as a consequence of irretrievable illness or injury, further therapy will not improve the patient's condition and, therefore, should not be attempted" [66]. Still, regardless of the circumstances, if the families are in a position to make decisions, they may demand the continuation of life-sustaining treatment, even if it may not be beneficial for the patient [67].

4.4 Examples

The relatives of a patient who receives end-of-life care may be emotionally overloaded, leaving them vulnerable to manipulation or driving them to manipulate the physicians. The most appropriate way to eliminate such manipulations from either party is medical ethical principles.

Patients and/or their families may be guided by a healthcare professional to seek a nonbeneficial, alternative treatment for an oncological disease that cannot be cured by modern medicine, and they may get false hopes regarding such treatments. They may even make catastrophic expenditures, using all their savings to seek such healthcare. This is quite a common example. Let us look at this example from the perspective of the four biomedical ethical principles. The patient and their families were not told the truth, and they were given incorrect information, which is against the principle of respect for autonomy and telling truth. The patient and their family were given false hope with methods that may harm them, which violates the principle of nonmaleficence and beneficence. The physician involved services that are not beneficial or evidence-based, which is against the principle of beneficence. Finally, the patient's chance to spend quality time with their loved ones was taken away, causing them to make catastrophic expenditures, which violates the principle of futility and beneficence.

A male patient did not respond to non-opioid analgesics and had pain and severe weight loss. He was diagnosed with incurable pancreatic cancer and was receiving PC at the hospital center. The patient's pain subsided after the opioid analgesic. The patient's daughter was in tears, worried that her father would become an opioid addict, so she wanted the opioid analgesics to be discontinued for 1 month. She also wanted to know if metastatic cancer in his liver grew, and therefore she requested radiological examinations. Believing that the demands made by the patient's daughter might be the patient's last wishes, the physician discontinued the opioid analgesics and ordered radiological imaging. Let us look at this example from the perspective of the four biomedical ethical principles. The physician discontinued the medication and requested radiological examinations without asking the patient's opinion, which violates the principle of respect for autonomy. The physician discontinued a drug that the patient was benefitting from, which is against the principle of beneficence. The physician caused more pain by discontinuing the drug, which violates the principle of nonmaleficence. Finally, the physician requested unnecessary radiological examination, which is against the principle of justice.

5. Conclusion

As a predecessor of bioethics and a branch of applied ethics, medical ethics was developed by physicians to regulate their interactions with their patients, colleagues, and society [68]. The patient-physician relationship is a unique interaction that is based on trust, dependency, and need, connecting the two [69]. This relationship is based on communication, ethical principles, and palliative care (PC); it differs from other clinics [3]. This is a stronger and more complex relationship that involves the PC team the patient, and the patient's family before death and during their grieving after death [3].

Laying down a set of rules that society expects medical physicians to abide by, the Hippocratic oath is a social contract with ethical principles [70]. The principles of medical ethics are taught intensively during the first years of medical faculties, but not adequately addressed after graduation, though they could be more useful during professional life [71].

The inevitability of death is highly likely to exert intense emotional pressure on the PC team, the patient, and the patient's families, including fear, hopelessness, despair, and anxiety. Dealing with this pressure appropriately is a part of good clinical management, but in doing so, ethical principles should not be compromised. Because they are not only a part of successful medical practice but a professional regulatory mechanism.

PC requires teamwork of doctors, nurses, physical therapists, clergy, and other essential health professionals [3]. Training the PC employees as a team both increases team communication and gives positive results in terms of patient safety [72]. Thus, the harm caused by communication to the patients and their families would be minimized.

The deaths witnessed by PC employees also affect their private lives [73]. Therefore, they must learn how to cope with the emotional burden of death and pain. Because they do a very special job, they should be trained on these issues. In this way, PC employees' tremendous emotional burdens would not hinder them from following their ethical principles and logic. Because PC principles should not be broken under the impact of emotions, treatments that are not evidence-based and are not beneficial to the patient should not be applied, and symptom management should not be considered secondary.

It is important to keep in mind that violating one principle of medical ethics may lead to a violation of others. The resources used for an unnecessary treatment for a patient in the PC may have violated the principles of truth-telling, respect for autonomy, nonmaleficence, beneficence, justice benefit, harm, justice, and futility.

Knowing, accepting, and applying ethical principles, even in the most unpleasant situations, provides a peaceful working environment for all employees.

Conflict of interest

The author declares no conflict of interest.

DOI: http://dx.doi.org/10.5772/intechopen.104990

Author details

Metin Dincer
Health Science Faculty, Department of Health Management, Ankara Yildirim Beyazit University, Ankara, Turkey

*Address all correspondence to: drmetindincer@yahoo.com

References

[1] Brennan F. Palliative care as an international human right. Journal of Pain and Symptom Management. 2007;**33**(5):494-499

[2] Kastbom L, Milberg A, Karlsson M. A good death from the perspective of palliative cancer patients. Support Care Cancer. 2017;**25**(3):933-939

[3] Connor SR, editor. Global Atlas of Palliative Care. 2nd ed. London: World Health Organization, Worldwide Palliative Care Alliance; 2020

[4] World Health Organization. Global Health and Aging. USA: NIH Publication [National Institute on Aging, National Institutes of Health, US Department of Health and Human Services]; 2011

[5] World Health Organization. Monitoring the Building Blocks of Health Systems: A Handbook of Indicators and their Measurement Strategies. Geneva, Switzerland: World Health Organization; 2010

[6] Hutter N, Stossel U, Meffert C, et al. "Good dying"—Definition and current state of research. Deutsche medizinische Wochenschrift (1946). 2015;**140**(17):1296-1301

[7] Cevizci A. Uygulamalı Etik. 2. Baskı ed. Say Yayınları: İstanbul; 2016

[8] Payne S, Lynch T. International progress in creating palliative medicine as a specialized discipline and the development of palliative care. Oxford Textbook of Palliative Medicine. 2015;**5**:3-9

[9] Wright M, Wood J, Lynch T, et al. Mapping levels of palliative care development: A global view. Journal of Pain and Symptom Management. 2008;**35**(5):469-485

[10] Clark D. Originating a movement: Cicely Saunders and the development of St. Christopher's Hospice, 1957-1967. Mortality. 1998;**3**(1):43-63

[11] Hui D, Nooruddin Z, Didwaniya N, et al. Concepts and definitions for "Actively Dying," "End of Life," "Terminally Ill," "Terminal Care," and "Transition of Care": A systematic review. Journal of Pain and Symptom Management. 2014;**47**(1):77-89

[12] End of Life Care. Available from: https://www.cancer.gov/publications/dictionaries/cancer-terms/def/end-of-life-care [Accessed: 15 March 2022]

[13] Dincer M, Kahveci K, Doger C. An examination of factors affecting the length of stay in a palliative care center. Journal of Palliative Medicine. 2018;**21**(1):11-15

[14] Wen F-H, Chen J-S, Chou W-C, et al. Family caregivers' subjective caregiving burden, quality of life, and depressive symptoms are associated with terminally ill cancer patients' distinct patterns of conjoint symptom distress and functional impairment in their last six months of life. Journal of Pain and Symptom Management. 2019;**57**(1):64-72

[15] Ferris FD, Bruera E, Cherny N, et al. Palliative cancer care a decade later: Accomplishments, the need, next steps—From the American Society of Clinical Oncology. Journal of Clinical Oncology. 2009;**27**(18):3052-3058

[16] Hsiu Chen C, Wen F-H, Hou M-M, et al. Transitions in prognostic awareness among terminally ill cancer patients in their last 6 months of life examined by multi-state Markov modeling. The Oncologist. 2017;**22**(9):1135-1142

[17] Bubis LD, Davis LE, Canaj H, et al. Patient-reported symptom severity among 22,650 cancer outpatients in the last six months of life. Journal of Pain and Symptom Management. 2020;**59**(1):58-66.e4

[18] World Health Organization. Cancer Pain Relief and Palliative Care: Report of a WHO Expert Committee [Meeting Held in Geneva from 3 to 10 July 1989]. Geneva: World Health Organization; 1990

[19] World Health Organization. Cancer Pain Relief and Palliative Care in Children. Geneva: World Health Organization; 1998

[20] Radbruch L, De Lima L, Knaul F, et al. Redefining palliative care—A new consensus-based definition. Journal of Pain and Symptom Management. 2020;**60**(4):754-764

[21] World Health Organization. Health Systems Strengthening Glossary. 2022 Avaible from: https://cdn.who.int/media/docs/defaultsource/documents/healthsystems-strengtheningglossary.pdf?sfvrsn=b871d95f_4. [Accessed: 2002-03-26]

[22] Tello J, Yelgezekova Z, Kruse I, et al. Glossary of Terms WHO European Primary Health Care Impact, Performance and Capacity Tool (PHC-IMPACT). Copenhagen Denmark: World Health Organization; 2019

[23] Beauchamp TL, Childress JF. Principles of Biomedical Ethics. 7th ed. New York, USA: Oxford University Press; 2013

[24] Kukla R. Conscientious autonomy: Displacing decisions in health care. The Hastings Center Report. 2005;**35**(2):34-44

[25] Culyer AJ, Newhouse JP, Pauly MV, et al. Handbook of Health Economics. The Netherlands: Elsevier; 2000

[26] Bickerdyke I, Dolamore R, Monday I, et al. Supplier-induced demand for medical services. In: Canberra: Productivity Commission Staff Working Paper. 2002. pp. 1-113

[27] Taylor RM. Ethical principles and concepts in medicine. Handbook of Clinical Neurology. 2013;**118**:1-9

[28] Barstow C, Shahan B, Roberts M. Evaluating medical decision-making capacity in practice. American Family Physician. 2018;**98**(1):40-46

[29] Howe EG. Beyond determining decision-making capacity. The Journal of Clinical Ethics. 2020;**31**(1):3-16

[30] Magnuson A, Mohile S, Janelsins M. Cognition and cognitive impairment in older adults with cancer. Current Geriatrics Reports. 2016;**5**(3):213-219

[31] Dinçer M. A retrospective study examining the properties and characteristics of dementia patients in a palliative care center. Turkish Journal of Medical Sciences. 2018;**48**(3):537-542

[32] Silveira MJ, Kim SY, Langa KM. Advance directives and outcomes of surrogate decision making before death. The New England Journal of Medicine. 2010;**362**(13):1211-1218

[33] Smith CM. Origin and uses of primum non nocere—Above all, do no harm! Journal of Clinical Pharmacology. 2005;**45**(4):371-377

[34] Gifford RW Jr. Primum non nocere. JAMA. 1977;**238**(7):589-590

[35] Institute of Medicine Committee on Data Standards for Patient Safety. In: Aspden P, Corrigan JM, Wolcott J, et al, editors. Patient Safety: Achieving a New Standard for Care. Washington, DC: National Academies Press; 2004

[36] Institute of Medicine Committee on Quality of Health Care in America.

In: Kohn LT, Corrigan JM, Donaldson MS, editors. To Err Is Human: Building a Safer Health System. Washington, DC: National Academies Press; 2000

[37] Makary MA, Daniel M. Medical error-the third leading cause of death in the US. BMJ. 2016;**353**:i2139

[38] Gillon R. Justice and medical ethics. British Medical Journal (Clinical Research Ed.). 1985;**291**(6489):201-202

[39] Avant LC, Swetz KM. Revisiting beneficence: What is a 'benefit', and by what criteria? The American Journal of Bioethics. 2020;**20**(3):75-77

[40] Sackett DL. Evidence-based medicine. Seminars in Perinatology. 1997;**21**(1):3-5

[41] OECD. Health Spending (Indicator). 2022. DOI: 10.1787/8643de7e-en. Available from: https://www.oecd-ilibrary.org/social-issues-migration-health/health-spending/indicator/english_8643de7e-en [Accessed: 26 March 2002]

[42] Capp S, Savage S, Clarke V. Exploring distributive justice in health care. Australian Health Review. 2001;**24**(2):40-44

[43] World Health Organization. Health Promotion Glossary of Terms. Geneva: World Health Organization; 2021

[44] World Health Organization. Health Equity Policy Tool: A Framework to Track Policies for Increasing Health Equity in the WHO European Region. Copenhagen, Denmark: World Health Organization, Regional Office for Europe; 2019

[45] Müller EC, Zimmermann J, Menzdorf L, et al. Medical confidentiality. Unfallchirurg. 2019;**122**(9):719-729

[46] Gillon R. Confidentiality. British Medical Journal (Clinical Research Ed.). 1985;**291**(6509):1634-1636

[47] Striegel H. Medical confidentiality in elite sports. Sportverletzung Sportschaden. 2018;**32**(1):61-65

[48] Surbone A. Truth telling. Annals of the New York Academy of Sciences. 2000;**913**:52-62

[49] Isaacs D. Telling the truth. Journal of Paediatrics and Child Health. 2016;**52**(6):585-586

[50] Zolkefli Y. The ethics of truth-telling in health-care settings. Malaysian Journal of Medical Sciences. 2018;**25**(3):135-139

[51] Whitney SN, Spiegel D. The patient, the physician, and the truth. The Hastings Center Report. 1999;**29**(3):24 [Discussion 24-5]

[52] Jones JW, McCullough LB, Richman BW. Truth-telling about terminal diseases. Surgery. 2005;**137**(3):380-382

[53] Martin J. Lying to patients: Can it ever be justified? Nursing Standard. 1993;**7**(18):29-31

[54] Benn P. Medicine, lies and deceptions. Journal of Medical Ethics. 2001;**27**(2):130-134

[55] Zwitter M. Dying and death. In: Zwitter M, editor. Medical Ethics in Clinical Practice. Cham: Springer International Publishing; 2019. pp. 127-135

[56] Wilkinson DJ, Savulescu J. Knowing when to stop: Futility in the ICU. Current Opinion in Anaesthesiology. 2011;**24**(2):160-165

[57] Derse AR. Limitation of treatment at the end-of-life: Withholding and

withdrawal. Clinics in Geriatric Medicine. 2005;**21**(1):223-238, xi

[58] Luce JM. Withholding and withdrawal of life support from critically ill patients. The Western Journal of Medicine. 1997;**167**(6):411-416

[59] Le Conte P, Riochet D, Batard E, et al. Death in emergency departments: A multicenter cross-sectional survey with analysis of withholding and withdrawing life support. Intensive Care Medicine. 2010;**36**(5):765-772

[60] van Beinum A, Hornby L, Ward R, et al. Variations in the operational process of withdrawal of life-sustaining therapy. Critical Care Medicine. 2015;**43**(10):e450-e457

[61] Mark NM, Rayner SG, Lee NJ, et al. Global variability in withholding and withdrawal of life-sustaining treatment in the intensive care unit: A systematic review. Intensive Care Medicine. 2015;**41**(9):1572-1585

[62] Lo B, Jonsen AR. Clinical decisions to limit treatment. Annals of Internal Medicine. 1980;**93**(5):764-768

[63] Whitmer M, Hurst S, Prins M, et al. Medical futility: A paradigm as old as hippocrates. Dimensions of Critical Care Nursing. 2009;**28**(2):67-71

[64] Cifrese L, Rincon F. Futility and patients who insist on medically ineffective therapy. Seminars in Neurology. 2018;**38**(5):561-568

[65] Trotter G. Mediating disputes about medical futility. Cambridge Quarterly of Healthcare Ethics. 1999;**8**(4):527-537

[66] Bernat JL. Medical futility. Neurocritical Care. 2005;**2**(2):198-205

[67] Schneiderman LJ, De Ridder M. Chapter 14 - Medical futility. In: Bernat JL, Beresford HR, editors. Handbook of Clinical Neurology. Vol. 118. Elsevier; 2013. pp. 167-179

[68] Baker R. Bioethics and history. The Journal of Medicine and Philosophy. 2002;**27**(4):447-474

[69] Veith I. Medical ethics throughout the ages. Quarterly Bulletin of Northwestern University Medical School. 1957;**31**(4):351-358

[70] Valentino M, Pavlica P. Medical ethics. Journal of Ultrasound. 2016;**19**(1):73-76

[71] Sokol D. When is the best time to teach medical ethics? BMJ. 2022;**376**:o504

[72] Conigliaro J. Teamwork and communication. In: Agrawal A, editor. Patient Safety: A Case-Based Comprehensive Guide. New York NY: Springer; 2014. pp. 19-33

[73] Dinçer M. Palyatif Bakım Hastalarına Resüsitasyon Uygulayan Sağlık Çalışanlarının Deneyimleri. The Experiences of Health Workers Applying Resuscitation to the Patients in Palliative Care. Ankara Medical Journal. 2019;**19**(1):21-31

Chapter 8

Palliative Care Therapies

Aisha Muthanna Shanshal

Abstract

Palliative care considered as a support care for anyone living with a complex disease such as cancer, it has a great role in decreasing the severity of illness and slowness loss of functions by symptoms control and management in different stages of cancer. Palliative care is a specialized care area bounded to deliver health care facilities to patients who suffer from direct, indirect symptoms, unmet needs, for prevention and relief suffering from psychological issues mainly emotional issues (depression, anxiety, and delirium) and physiological issues like (nausea, vomiting, fatigue, xerostomia, headache, osteoradionecrosis, hemoptysis, dyspnea, taste loss, and pain). So its goal is to prolong their survival with the best possible quality of life for both the patients and their families.

Keywords: palliative care, cancer, symptoms, quality of life

1. Introduction

Cancer considers the first cause of death globally and it is accounting for about 10 million deaths in 2020 [1]. It has bad impact on physical and social life. Patients with cancer may experience one symptom or more at one time. Those with advanced disease that characterized by breathlessness and metastatic cancer may have on average about 14 symptoms [2], including symptoms of cancer itself and the side effect of cancer therapies [3].

Non-curative therapy creates a multidisciplinary effort for patients whose disease is unresponsive to indicated treatment curative intent, so its purpose is life-enhancing and prolonging. Those patients will go through progressive disease, that makes patients suffer from restlessness as a result of their illness, strategies of treatment, which negatively affect their treatment and the recovering handle, so, it is fundamental to control and reduce such suffering, which makes them need a shift in the objective of medical care. Despite the fact, that life-prolonging treatment can provide prolonged disease control with the present armamentarium of treatment modalities, side effects such as pain, anxiety, depression, fatigue, dyspnea, diarrhea, loss of appetite, nausea, and vomiting, often reduce the patient's quality of life [4–8].

In order to prevent/palliate these negative impacts of the outcomes of the disease and to enhance quality of life of patients and their families, the urgency for palliative care as the main goal in providing therapy and care for patients who face problems of life-threatening diseases. Palliative care can relieve of the patient's suffering by early identification, evaluation and treatment of physical, psychological, and social problems that include request for hastened death, assistance with making decision or care planning, patient demand for referral, spinal cord compression, delirium, brain, or leptomeningeal metastases [9–13].

According to the World Health Organization (WHO), more than 50% of the countries in the world are making efforts to provide treatment and palliative care for cancer patients. At the same time, many countries do not have a cancer control program [14]. Approximated cancer patients require more than one-quarter of global palliative care need [15]. Lack of enough communication enhance stress, decrease patient satisfaction, and decrease strictly following medical instructions, so adequate collection of data at a palliative care service enhance quality of patient care [16–18]. Early appearance of palliative care enhances quality of life, decreases therapeutic cost, and superior survival time. But, to provide convenient care to cancer patients, it is necessary to refer them to health services timely [19].

The core focus of palliative care also improves the care quality for the health care system [20, 21]. Besides improving physical symptoms, it will reduce emergency visits and reduces hospital admissions. For patients who have not taken palliative care at all or who came late to palliative care are more probably to receive invasive treatments, such as chemotherapy, and increase risk of death from treatment complications. Starting the palliative care at the time of diagnosis provides an adjuvant partnership for the treatment team and as the disease develops, the need for palliative care increases. That's why it is suggested that palliative care be started in the first 8 weeks after the onset of the disease and the American Society of Oncology Guidelines also suggested that palliative care be initiated at the onset of cancer for some patients [22–25].

That's can improve all phases of the disease, it makes better decisions in the end-of-life care and potentially decreases health-care expenditures [26], and can generate consequential savings for the health system by decreasing hospitalization and interventions [27].

2. Palliative care for lung cancer patients

Lung cancer is considered as the main cause of cancer death among both men and women in the world [28]. The survival rate is estimated not more than 5-year [29] and the average survival patients who do not take any anti-neoplastic treatment is about 7 months, according to a meta-analysis of over 5000 patients [30]. The main reasons of death from lung cancer included complications of metastases, tumor burden, infection, thromboembolism, pulmonary hemorrhage, and diffuse alveolar damage. The final common attributor for most of these complications is respiratory failure. Both survivals, quality of life and symptoms are commonly worse for patients with end stage of the disease. Symptoms related to lung cancer can include pain, anorexia/cachexia, dyspnea, nausea, fatigue, confusion/delirium, and depression [31].

As pain is generally part of the reasons behind the suffering in these patients, beside psychological distress. Opioids are chief support that provides effective analgesia in cancer pain, such as morphine, which considered as is the most used opioid for moderate to severe pain. It can be used rectally or transdermally in patients who cannot take it orally [32]. Low-dose corticosteroids are also recommended for relieving pain from liver metastases, bony metastases, or neuropathic pain [33]. Anticonvulsants such as phenytoin, carbamazepine, and clonazepam are also helpful in treating that pain. Tricyclic antidepressants increase the effects of opioids and have analgesic properties [34].

Other symptoms that can develop from locally advanced NSCLC or lung cancer metastases are dyspnea and cough, these symptoms are disease-related complications, such as malignant effusions and airway obstruction. Therapeutic procedures with palliative aide can be helpful, such as pericardiocentesis with a pericardial drain/window, thoracentesis, or placement of pleural drain [35]. Other strategies for resolving airway obstruction include laser therapy, bronchoscopy, stent placement (endobronchial or vascular), or photodynamic therapy [36].

Morphine is usually used drug while recommendation of codeine or dihydrocodeine may be considered in dyspnea with lower intensity [37, 38]. Other opioids, including fentanyl and oxycodone, have been studied in this management, opioid mechanism of action is conveyed via opioid receptors of the cardio-respiratory system [39]. Benzodiazepines are also utilized as an adjunct, or as an alternative, to opioids for treating dyspnea which considered as a second or third choice in cases where morphine and non-pharmacological methods are not enough to control dyspnea [40]. Anticholinergic drugs such as hyoscyamine, scopolamine, atropine, and glycopyrrolate can be described to decrease excessive secretions [41, 42].

In 47–86% of lung cancer patients, cough is one of the most common symptoms of lung cancer. Pharmacotherapy includes administration of antitussive drugs and opioids. Oral corticosteroids that are taken for 14 days may resolve coughing result from direct infiltration of the bronchus by the tumor. As consequences of cough, gastrointestinal reflux may occur; which may resolve with metoclopramide or domperidone. Dihydrocodeine, codeine also can be prescribed as antitussive opioid, codeine is usually in complex preparations with paracetamol. Constipation on the other hand is a complication of systematic administration of opioid, therefore prophylactic administration of laxatives is essential. Morphine or other strong opioids such as methadone are recommended for severe cough with pain in the chest, co-administration of more than one opioid is not appropriate. Mucolytic agents such as bromhexine and acetylcysteine that can be taken orally or by inhalation, but have limited use [43, 44].

Hemoptysis is a symptom that appears in about 20% of lung cancer patients. Pulmonary hemorrhage, which usually leads to death, is noticed in 3% of patients. The reasons behind hemoptysis include bronchiectasis, trauma after bronchoscopy, anticoagulation therapy, pulmonary embolism, fistulas, and others. Tranexamic acid and medications that support hemostasis such as vitamin K and antitussives are drugs that inhibit fibrinolysis that is used in adjunctive therapy at the end stage of disease. Also in the mentioned stage of disease mitigation procedures are used such as an appropriate position to forbid choking, taking anti-anxiety drugs (diazepam, midazolam) and using bed linen in dark colors [37, 43] in case of superior vena cava syndrome. The most seen symptoms include swelling of the face and congestion, upper chest and shoulders, shortness of breath, hoarseness, fainting on standing at the slope, dizziness, headache, and extension veins in the neck and the chest wall, corticosteroids such as dexamethasone are used as palliative treatment. Also, the use of heparin because of risk of thrombosis SVCS in the superior vena cava is reasonable [43, 45, 46].

Nutrition and appetite stimulants advising can be considered for patients with critical appetite and weight loss. Low-dose corticosteroids for appetite stimulation are unclear, but the benefit of it is often related to its antiemetic effect. Medications such as stimulants, antidepressants, steroids, and erythropoietin-stimulating agents have been assessed for treating fatigue but without definite evidence of benefit. The intervention studied for enhancing fatigue is exercise and physical activity [47–49].

3. Palliative care for ovarian cancer patients

Generally, it is called as the silent killer and it is the dominant gynecological cancer worldwide. Long-term survival of more than 5 years for those with advanced disease is realized in approximately 25% of patients [50–52]. Ovarian cancer's early-stage signs and symptoms are usually vague and similar to other genitourinary or gastrointestinal illnesses. The recurrence is about 70% of ovarian cancer patients. Nearly all of the parenteral cytotoxic drugs indicated for recurrent ovarian cancer have massive side effects that decrease the therapeutic benefit and consequently patients' acceptance of therapy. The less toxic alternative is altretamine which works to enhance the outcome of these patients.

Altretamine is an oral alkylating activity drug that has been prescribed for advanced ovarian carcinoma, it is prescribed for patients with recurrent ovarian cancer or who had undergone surgery and failed one or more chemotherapy regimen. It works as palliation for those with recurrent disease or as a maintenance drug to enhance and increase progression-free survival for these patients. Most benefit of altretamine is the decrease of physical and psychological discomfort came with the parenteral therapies and its oral use decreases the need for hospitalization [53, 54].

Besides altretamine, palliative therapy is used to minimize the symptoms of ovarian cancer. Women with ovarian cancer can have *ascites*. It can be very annoying but can be treated with *paracentesis*. It is a procedure where skin is numbed, a needle is inserted to withdraw the fluid. Another therapeutic option is a catheter which placed into the abdomen and the fluid can be eliminated as often as is needed. Bevacizumab (Avastin) can also help by slow fluid buildup, it is injected directly into the abdomen. These treatments can decrease symptoms, but rarely, might aide some women live longer. After all, their effects are temporary, and the cancer persists.

Another symptom is intestinal tract *obstruction*. That can cause nausea, vomiting, and abdominal pain, another procedure to allow the stomach juices to drain so that the digestive tract isn't completely blocked, this is done by placing a tube through the skin and into the stomach [55, 56]. Other therapies to facilitate bowel movements include, drinking adequate fluids, and gentle exercise. To manage the symptoms of constipation some medications can be prescribed including ondansetron as anti-emitting, Miralax as laxatives, and steroids to reduce inflammation [57].

3.1 Pelvic or abdominal pain

At the beginning of ovarian cancer, pain can be easily ignored, hard to diagnose, or missed with other conditions. But, later in advance stage of ovarian cancer, it may cause a lot of pain and discomfort in the abdominal parts of your body. Over-the-counter (OTC) pain medications such as acetaminophen or anti-inflammatory pain relievers ibuprofen (Motrin, Advil). If your pain isn't controlled by OTC medications, an opioid indicated in such cases, can help minimize stronger pain such as morphine, fentanyl patch, hydromorphone, and methadone. Also find an alternative therapy to decrease abdominal pain, for example, massage, try: acupuncture, relaxation techniques, such as guided imagery, meditation, and chiropractic treatment.

Ovarian cancer can expand and affect the urinary system. Its tumor can block the ureters that prevent the urine from reaching the bladder, which results in swelling, pain, and kidney damage if don't treat. To relieve this pressure and pain, a special tube may utilize to drain the urine during cancer treatment. The tube can be placed inside the body to excrete urine from the kidney into the bladder, or outside of the body to excrete urine directly from the kidney.

Bloating and swelling can be seen at any stage of ovarian cancer. OTC remedies may not decrease this discomfort; octreotide may decrease these symptoms. Additionally, decreasing secondary bloating by staying away from carbonated beverages, processed foods, and gas-producing foods such as cabbage, beans, and broccoli [58–61].

4. Palliative care for metastatic bone cancer patients

The skeletal system is the third most known site for cancer metastases, particularly in end stages of the disease. The presence of bone metastases leads to poorer diagnosis, decrease of survival and is usually associated with several complications, including spinal cord compression, severe bone pain, pathological fracture, and hypercalcemia, etc. [62–65]. Nearly 60–84% of patients with late cancer experiences varying level of bone pain. Bon pain affects millions of patients worldwide, and approximately 450,000 patients in the USA alone annually [66, 67]. Generally, pain varies in severity depending on the stage of the disease. Most patients at the beginning of the disease experience infrequent dull aches, but as the disease advanced, pain becomes constant and increase in severity [68, 69].

Analgesic medications involve pain management with analgesics (non-opioid and opioid), adjuvants (corticosteroids, anticonvulsants), and bone-targeted therapies (NGF inhibitors; osteoclast inhibitors, such as denosumab and bisphosphonates). Radiotherapy (RT) is also used to reduce analgesic need, enhance the quality of life (QoL), also keep or improve skeletal function by minimizing the risk of metastatic spinal cord compression (mSCC) or pathological fractures [70].

Bone-seeking radiopharmaceuticals emitting-particles such as [223Ra] radium-dichloride at the top have been prescribed for bone-pain palliation. Beside [223Ra] a number of long-established and novel bone-seeking radiopharmaceuticals are prescribed for bone-pain palliation, including [89Sr] strontium-dichloride, [153Sm] samarium, [186Re] rhenium, [188Re] rhenium, [177Lu] lutetium, and [166Ho] holmium labeled [71–76]. the control of painful bone metastases is still a challenging problem. Bone-pain palliation with radiopharmaceuticals emitting-particles been utilized for decades, demonstrate an acceptable result. [223Ra] Radium shows higher advantages impact on survival over other radiopharmaceuticals; at the same time, still the expensive [223Ra] radium is not generally available [77].

5. Palliative care for pancreatic cancer patients

Pancreatic cancer is the twelfth most common cancer in the world and the seventh leading cause of cancer death. It has a poor survival rate, it mortality rate about 4.0% of all cancer deaths [78–80]. Now a day surgical resection is the only choice for treatment, however, only 20% of pancreatic cancer is surgically removable at the time of diagnosis [81–83]. The maximum survival rates are 22–26 months in patients who are undergoing surgical resection and taking adjuvant therapy resect able to improve survival [84–87] latest studies evaluating the effect of neoadjuvant therapy on highly picked patients with resect able disease have led to median survival life about 44 months in patients with R0 resection, node-negative disease [88–90].

5.1 Planned operative and endoscopic palliation

Choledochojejunostomy or Roux-en-Y hepatico was surgical palliation that was most commonly done. But its performance fell out of favor as a result of a high probability of cystic duct, gastric outlet, or duodenal obstruction by the tumor over time, as well as the likelihood of bile reflux into the stomach. The placing of endoscopic biliary stents throughout endoscopic retrograde cholangiopancreatography (ERCP) is the favorite method for palliation of obstructive jaundice in patients with metastatic or unresectable pancreatic cancer. Development in endoscopic technology results in successful stent placement in more than 90% of patients during ERCP with the same efficacy, but less mortality and morbidity in comparison with surgical palliation with biliary-enteric bypass. After all, studies still present the majority of patients who are stented have an enhancement in quality of life, even with higher rates of recurrence [91–93]. Prophylactic gastrojejunostomy was associated with a diminished incidence of late GOO (gastric outlet obstruction). It was also indicated in patients with unresectable periampullary cancer that undergo exploratory laparotomy [94–96].

5.2 Endoscopic palliation

Treatment of gastric outlet obstruction can be done endoscopically, with placing of large self-expanding stents which are successful in 92–100% of cases permitting patients to take back oral intake in 24 hours in 73–93% of patients. Even though patients can control their own drink liquids and salivary secretions, stent obstruction usually occurs with solid food [91, 93].

5.3 Thromboembolic disease

Pancreatic cancer patients have one of the highest frequencies of pulmonary embolism (PE) or deep venous thrombosis (DVT) with incidence rates between 17 and 57%. Anticoagulation drugs with low-molecular-weight heparin or a direct oral anticoagulant are useful in patients who develop a VTE. Many studies estimate this risk, showing a 10–25% risk of VTE, with minimization to 5–10% with thromboprophylaxis but no effect on survival. Treatment includes treatment with low weight molecular heparin (LWMH), unfractionated heparin, or oral anticoagulation [97].

6. Palliative care for oral cancer patients

Patients may experience oral side effects as a result of disease or medications. Anti-cancer medications have acute and long-term adverse effects on healthy tissue. The epithelium of the oral mucosa can be affected by most therapeutic agents that may cause xerostomia, mucositis, and taste alterations [98–105].

Beside this side effect, patients in the end stage of the disease, perhaps as a result of their weakness, oral symptoms are one of their highest sources of discomfort. Symptoms involve oral candidiasis, angular cheilitis, oral pain, mucositis, denture stomatitis, dysphagia, ulceration, taste disorders, oral infection, halitosis, and dry mouth, which is the most familiar oral symptom. The causes behind oral problems are several, such as general weakness from disease or its medications; previous cancer treatment, such as chemotherapy and radiotherapy; dehydration; and the decrease

DOI: http://dx.doi.org/10.5772/intechopen.105220

the ability of water or food intake; their physical condition may decay because of oral symptoms, which lead to inability of food intake and dehydration [106–109].

7. Oral care palliative care protocol

At the beginning of oral care, a facial massage of the masseter muscle and salivary glands. An oral moisture jelly and moisture spray were utilized for enhancing mucosal moisture and for protecting the mucosa. Also, a soft dental brush was used to remove plaque and debris on the teeth. Then, oral foam sticks were utilized for mucosa cleansing [110].

Palliative treatment for squamous cell carcinoma treatment included mono-chemotherapy with the administration of cetuximab. The side effects of cetuximab are manageable. The common reactions are mostly cutaneous, with the appearance of acne, dryness, itching, and peeling on the skin [111]. Corticosteroids such as prednisone are usually administrated with the cetuximab treatment to minimize the previously mentioned adverse effects. Nonetheless, the repeated use of this medication may cause other disturbances, such as osteoporosis [112].

7.1 Pain management for oral cancer patients

Cancer pain may result from direct invasion cell of cancer into the nerve or bone tissue in the end stages of oral cancer and its management is critical issue [113]. Opioid analgesics are usually prescribed for controlling oral cancer-related pain. In spite of high dosages of opioids are prescribed, high level of cancer pain is usually poorly controlled. Switching is often necessary due to different side effects or tolerance of opioids. Methadone has been widely prescribed to manage oral pain because of its exclusive properties (e.g., long duration of action strong, high bioavailability, and analgesic effect) [114].

7.2 Xerostomia prevention therapies

Xerostomia is one of common adverse effects of radiation therapy on salivary glands. Radiation exposure may change saliva volume, consistency, and its pH. The inadequate saliva can decrease the quality of life as the patient cannot carry forward with his routine diet, which came with difficulty in swallowing and dysguesia that can lead to nutrition deficiency. Several managements are utilized to decrease xerostomia such as water-soluble lubricants that must be applied thinly over the oral mucosal surfaces to lubricate the oral tissues. Mouth rinses that contain alcohol should not be used in such cases as they will increase mouth dryness.

Salivary stimulation agents should be advised, like vitamin C and citric acids, sugar free topical agents malic acid that used topically can stimulate saliva, though, their low pH enhances demineralization of teeth. Salivary stimulation agent proves to be beneficial for the xerostomia patient and should be taken before eating to enhance swallowing. The two most common pharmacologic medications prescribed to stimulate salivary secretion are cholinergic agonists such as cevimiline and pilocarpine, treatment continues for 12 weeks of uninterrupted therapy is recommended. These drugs are contraindicated in patients with narrow-angle glaucoma, acute iritis, and asthmatic patient [115, 116].

Bethanechol chloride cholinergic agonist that its works in contrast to acetylcholine, bethanechol has more prolonged effects as a result of resistant to destruction by cholinesterase. Its mechanism of action is similar to pilocarpine, stimulating the parasympathetic nervous system. It acts more specifically on the muscarinic receptors, not acting on α/β-adrenergic receptors, as pilocarpine does [117]. These medications work as systemic stimulants of salivary gland acting on the parasympathetic nervous system. The response to enhance salivation is depending on the residual number of functional acinar cells [118].

Herbal medicines were also found to enhance salivary function and to decrease the severity of mouth dryness in cancer patients [119]. In spite of several RCTs of acupuncture as a management for dry mouth have been stated to date, its cumulative evidence for its effectiveness has not been systematically estimatted [120]. An organic thiophosphate is amifostine that can protect cells from radiation distruction by scavenging oxygen-derived free radicals. The prescription of amifostine is very controversial because of its toxicity, cost, and compromised tumor control, in spite of all previous disadvantages, it is considered the only drug approved by FDA for xerostomia result from radioprotection [121]. The prophylactic use of systemic sialogogues for radiation-induced xerostomia is widely reported in the literature [122].

7.3 Management of taste loss and candidiasis

Chemotherapy and radiotherapy for oral cancer can change or reduce taste function as a result of the outer surface of taste cells and microvilli and damage that leads to limitation in food intake and weight loss as consequences. Taste loss is generally temporary and returns gradually to normal levels within 1 year after taking radiotherapy but sometimes it may last for 5 years [123]. High incidence of non-Candida albicans infection has been estimated in patients with end stage of cancer. The untreated colonized Candida can lead to disseminated disease that can end with morbidity and mortality. Fluconazole is considered as one of the first-line medications prescribed for management of oral candidiasis in cancer patients. Amphotericin B and newer drugs like echinocandins are also used for invasive Candida infections [124, 125].

Taste is very important for life; it manages food intake and provides pleasure feeling from eating. The taste regulates digestion, absorption, and storage of nutrient perception by activation neuronal pathways [126]. Alteration or taste dysfunction (dysgeusia) may decrease the quality of life by affecting and psychological well-being, appetite, and body weight. Several factors can affect taste perception, such as lesions in the oral mucosa, medication, prolonged exposure to radiation and chemotherapy, smoking, nutrition, chronic hepatitis, aging, renal impairment, and disorder in hormonal secretions [127]. Zinc supplements can be useful for patients receiving chemotherapy. Zinc protected the cancer patients from taste alteration [128] other form, a zinc containing polaprezinc that can also protect against taste disorder [129]. Amifostine, protect salivary gland normal tissues from damage by chemotherapy and radiation [130] thus leading to improvement of xerostomia that may cause taste alterations [131].

7.4 Osteoradionecrosis

Osteoradionecrosis is a complication result from radiation therapy to the head and neck that results in bone death, its side effect includes neuropathic pain [132]. Hyperbaric oxygen (HBO) therapy companied surgery can be used in the management of osteoradionecrosis, HBO enhances tissue oxygenation through control of infection, angiogenesis, predominantly through stimulate bacterial killing fungi, macrophages, and production of bactericidal free radicals [133, 134]. Other treatment modalities—Ultrasound has reported to stimulate tissue regeneration by enhancing blood flow in chronically ischemic muscles, protein synthesis and cure of ischaemic varicose ulcers. Pentoxifylline and calcitonin also have been used successfully to treat ORN [135].

7.5 Psychological and other factors

Antiemetics such as selective serotonin type 3 receptor (5HT3) antagonists (e.g., ondansetron, granisetron), neurokinin 1 receptor antagonists (e.g., fosaprepitant, aprepitant), and synthetic cannabinoids (e.g., nabilone) are licensed for use in chemotherapy-induced nausea and vomiting (CINV) [136]. In response to oral cancer treatment there may be changes in patients including their ability to swallow, speech, taste deprivation of sleep or metabolic disorders, and alterations in appearance. These changes can be emotionally harmful to the patient. This required psychiatric interventions in such patients.

8. Palliative care in head and neck cancer

Cancer of head and neck is the sixth most common cancer, the overall survival rate is 5-year that has ranged from 40 to 65%, affected by several factors such as co-morbidities and advanced-stage disease presentation [137, 138].

8.1 Surgical palliation

Incurable end-stage head and neck cancer lead to upsetting symptoms such as pain, bleeding, swallowing, and breathing difficulty. Patients may try to stay active and self-caring while trying to adapt to these symptoms. Surgery can decrease primary tumor bulk, decrease pain and bleeding, enhance swallowing, nutrition and airway, many evidence is available to estimate the surgical benefit in such cases. Also, an endovascular technique, involving embolization and vessel stenting, can help by controlling bleeding symptoms result from major vascular erosion. However, benzodiazepines are rapid-acting sedatives that reduce the flow of blood with direct pressure that administrated when patient succumbs rapidly in case of acute hemorrhage from carotid "blow-out." Whilst success may achieve with swift surgical intervention, continuous verbal support to the patient is a key to control and decrease anxiety. Besides benzodiazepines, use of bisphosphonates aid pain control of bone pain.

8.2 Pain

Pain is very familiar symptom that affects patients at any stage of cancer. It can be immediate or persistent lifelong. Analgesic use is the preferred one based on the WHO. Choice of formulation depends on patient conditions, if he can swallow. Persist vomiting has a nasogastric or gastrostomy tube. In case of somatic pain, oral morphine is the first choice strong opioid such as Oramorph™ solution or Sevredol™ tablet (e.g., MST Continus™) or capsules (e.g., Zomorph™) and suspension (e.g., MST suspension™) or opened capsules (e.g., Zomorph™).

In case of continuous vomiting, subcutaneous (SC) infusion of morphine or diamorphine can be prescribed such as diamorphine, transdermal preparations of fentanyl. Alternatively, new formulations of sublingual, buccal, or intranasal fentanyl may have a role in specific situations. Oxycodone may act as an alternative to morphine when there is intolerance, specifically dysphoria, the injected form of hydromorphone is useful. Liquid form of methadone in can be very useful, because of its rapidity in onset and long acting.

Neuropathic pain is a very common feature of the disease and also can result from treatment, specially radiation. Some medications can be referred to as adjuvants such as a tricyclic antidepressants (e.g., amitriptyline), anticonvulsants (gabapentin and pregabalin). Gabapentin in some cases opened and administered via the gastrostomy tube. Also carbamazepine, sodium valproate also can be used. Clonazepam is sometimes useful. Methadone and ketamine are useful, but only in specific settings. In case of visceral pain, if the pain is poorly sensitive to opioids, adjuvants should be administrated early, for example, pain due to nerve compression or metastatic disease in the liver cab is controlled with dexamethasone (4–8 mg daily). Interventional pain techniques may be very useful when systemic treatments fail or in case the patient is intolerant of the significant doses of analgesics combination.

In case of mucosal pain topical agents can be used such as chlorhexidine, sulcralfate, benzydamine, steroids, and topical local anaesthetics such as lignocaine. High number of patients who are enterally fed suffer from nausea and vomiting, so there is usually a need for injectable anti-emetics—continuous infusions, subcutaneous (SC), or boluses. Enteral feeding has its own challenge; prokinetic drugs like metoclopramide or domperidone may be utilized to establish the best function.

8.3 Constipation

Constipation develops in 50% of cancer patients as a result of decreased physical activity, dehydration, hypercalcemia, hypothyroidism, and some kind of medications, specially opioids and anticholinergic drugs. Laxatives can be stated once opioid medication is initiated. Laxative agents include bisacodyl, senna, lactulose, magnesium hydroxide, docusate, movicol, laxido. If constipation develops it can lead to nausea and vomiting and in the severe situations pseudo-obstruction. If rectal examination reveals hard stool, then the use of suppositories and enemas can be helpful.

8.4 Anxiety

Benzodiazepines are the main treatment of anxiety. Such as diazepam, lorazepam, and midazolam. However, the limiting point is developing tolerance very fast; so they are useful only for short-term control of episodes of anxiety.

8.5 Delirium

Delirium is a neuropsychiatric condition that is may increase incidence of morbidity and mortality in patients with end stage disease, which profoundly impacts the patients, their families, and their caregivers [139]. As a cause of confusion can result from number of organic causes such as metabolic disturbance, respiratory failure, infection, dehydration, urinary retention, constipation, brain metastases, and other causes. Common causes are administered drugs specially opioids.

Usually, delirium is controlled with haloperidol or levomepromazine where sedation is required for managing paranoia. In some conditions, like irreversible agitation or delirium in end stage patients, benzodiazepines and antipsychotics are required to administered together using a syringe driver secretions [9]. The most common used antipsychotic drugs in delirium patients are phenothiazines (e.g., chlorpromazine), butyrophenones (e.g., haloperidol), second-generation antipsychotics (e.g., olanzapine, risperidone, quetiapine, and ziprasidone), and third-generation antipsychotics (e.g., aripiprazole). In spite of little supporting data, there is no approved medication for delirium, antipsychotics are widely used but still the role of antipsychotics remains uncertain [140–144]. Excess secretions at the end stage of cancer are treated using anticholinergic medication to support this end-of-life phase. Also, there are three widely used antimuscarinic drugs that can be prescribed for excess secretion which include hyoscine hydrobomide, hyoscine butylbromide, and glycopyrronium [9].

9. Palliative care for colorectal cancer patients

Colorectal cancer is the third most common malignant disease about 1.85 million of new cases a year around the world and nearly 10.2% of total [145]. Surgical resection may consider as good palliation of symptoms and prevent harmful complications consequences [146].

10. Palliative care for bladder cancer patients

Bladder cancer is the ninth most common malignancy in the world [147]. The 5-year survival for bladder cancer is 76.9%, however, metastatic disease 5-year survival rate is only 5.5% [148]. It is mainly seen in elderly people [149]. Bladder cancer can cause persistent and disabling pain in patients [150] pelvic pain is one of the major end-of-life complications in people suffering from bladder cancer [151]. The pain control in some cases was adequate with fentanyl patches [152] bleeding can also arise from the bladder cancer, or as a result of radiation or cyclophosphamide, infection can also worsen bleeding. Patients with severe haematuria can be treated with palliative TURBT, tranexamic acid, palliative radiotherapy, embolisation, palliative chemotherapy, and urinary diversion [153].

11. Palliative care for breast cancer patients

Breast cancer is the most common cancer among women worldwide and the most common cause of cancer death in women. About 23% of the 1.1 million female with cancers newly diagnosed every year. And about one-fifth will survive for 5 years; American Cancer Society estimated that breast cancer is the second only to lung cancer as a cause of cancer death in women [154–159].

11.1 Pain

In general, the major causes of cancer-related pain in breast cancer women are bone metastases [160, 161]. Opioid analgesic medications can be submitted for patients with strong pain, in the case of neuropathic patient, patients may get benefit by combined analgesic with an agent with special efficacy for this mechanism of pain like tricyclic, SNRI, and/or an anticonvulsant. Radiotherapy may be also important in case of bone metastases for patients with poorly controlled pain [161–163].

11.2 Breathlessness (dyspnea)

Patients with breast cancer usually suffer from breathlessness; there are many causes of dyspnea and for its management, non-pharmacological and pharmacological approaches can be used [39]. Sitting the patient in upright position, use of bedside relaxation techniques, and accelerating air flow over the face using a fan or open window, are all helpful. Also, large symptomatic pericardial or pleural effusions should be drained. Oxygen supplementation can decrease dyspnea for patients with hypoxemia. Opioids are also approved for symptomatic therapy for dyspnea at the end stage of the disease [164].

11.3 Fatigue

Fatigue is the most common cause of distress to the patients. Restoration of energy strategies involved taking adequate nutrition and rest, decreasing stress can be done by several techniques like meditation or relaxation. Physical exercise proved to be useful in many clinical trials [165]. Fatigue patient's anemia with a hemoglobin of lower than 8 g/dL may require blood transfusion to maintain a hemoglobin level between 10 and 12 g/dL. Some studies mentioned that methylphenidate or modafanil can be useful for patient with fatigue symptoms but till now there are some limited data about its benefits regarding fatigue [166]. Steroids may have a role in short-term control or decease of fatigue for a patient who needs to be in his optimal alertness for an important family event or special occasion, but there is no benefit in long-term fatigue management [164].

11.4 Depression

Patient having cancer can be depressed experience, its incidence lower than anxiety. Although, it can be underreported by patients [167, 168]. Depression in cancer patients usually needs combining antidepressant medications, supportive psychotherapy, and cognitive-behavioral techniques [169]. Antidepressant is the main management for cancer patients with severe depressive symptoms that should be accompanied by psychotherapy by a professional therapist. That include selective serotonin re-uptake inhibitors (e.g., fluoxetine, sertraline, paroxetine, citalopram, and fluvoxamine), serotonin-norepinephrine reuptake inhibitor (e.g., venlaflaxine), and the serotonin-2 antagonists'/serotonin reuptake inhibitors, nefazodone and trazodone, and psychostimulants (e.g., methylphenidate) [170].

However, home palliative care enhances care and rehabilitation, its practiced by the interdisciplinary team help the patient to stay at home, in familiar environment, where relaxation and comfort not founded in the environment of the hospital. Necessary equipment is brought home to conduct therapy, such as an infusion pump. From time to time, qualified medical personnel should visit the patients allow efficient communications with patients and their families, manage the therapy, checking bedsores, and explain proceedings in the case of unexpected health hazards. For patients who cannot be medically managed at home, staying in inpatient care units for control or alleviate the symptoms is not adequate or sufficient [171].

12. Conclusion

This study summarized different kinds of palliative therapies for different types of cancer that improves the wellbeing of patients with life-limiting condition. It supports their families by identification patient needs, correct assessment and use of therapeutics for control health-related concerns such as management of physical issues (reliving patient from pain) and dealing with psychosocial, emotional state. Early palliative care prolongs life by decreasing morbidity and improved quality of life by using different strategies which include medication, surgical, nutrition, and home palliative care. It also reduces the load, strain of hospital related stresses and unnecessary hospital visits, in addition to decreasing hospital and health care cost.

Author details

Aisha Muthanna Shanshal
Al-Rafidain University College, Baghdad, Iraq

*Address all correspondence to: rafeef_sh@yahoo.com

References

[1] Ferlay J, Ervik M, Lam F, Colombet M, Mery L, Piñeros M, et al. Global Cancer Observatory: Cancer Today. Vol. 17. Lyon, France: International Agency for Research on Cancer; 2018. pp. 1-6

[2] Bausewein C, Booth S, Gysels M, et al. Understanding breathlessness: Cross-sectional comparison of symptom burden and palliative care needs in chronic obstructive pulmonary disease and cancer. Journal of Palliative Medicine. 2010;**13**:1109-1118

[3] Patrick D, Ferketich S, Frame P, et al. National Institutes of Health state of the science conference statement: Symptom management in cancer: Pain, depression and fatigue. Journal of the National Cancer Institute. Monographs. 2004;**32**:9-16

[4] Jacobsen PB, Andrykowski MA. Tertiary prevention in cancer care: Understanding and addressing the psychological dimensions of cancer during the active treatment period. The American Psychologist. 2015;**70**(2):134

[5] Teunissen SC, Wesker W, Kruitwagen C, de Haes HC, Voest EE, de Graeff A. Symptom prevalence in patients with incurable cancer: A systematic review. Journal of Pain and Symptom Management. 2007;**34**(1):94-104

[6] Hessissen L, Kili A. Palliative care in Moroccan children with cancer: What are the parent's and children's needs? Palliative Medicine and Hospice Care – Open Journal. 2017;**SE(1)**:S56-S583

[7] Higginson IJ, Evans CJ. What is the evidence that palliative care teams improve outcomes for cancer patients and their families? The Cancer Journal. 2010;**16**(5):423-435

[8] Bruera E, Yennurajalingam S. Palliative care in advanced cancer patients: How and when? The Oncologist. 2012;**17**(2):267-273

[9] Cocks H, Ah-See K, Capel M, Taylor P. Palliative and supportive care in head and neck cancer: United Kingdom National Multidisciplinary Guidelines. The Journal of Laryngology & Otology. 2016;**130**(S2):S198-S207

[10] World Health Organization. Definition of Palliative Care. 2008. Available from: http://www.who.int/cancer/palliative/definition/en/ [Accessed: 27 July 2015]

[11] Ghafoor I, Hafeez H, Naz F, Baker MA. Comparison of documented patient care before and after implementation of end of life care pathway for terminally ill patients at Shaukat Khanum Memorial Cancer Hospital and Research Centre. Journal of Cancer & Allied Specialties. 2018;**4**(3)

[12] Yamaguchi T, Kuriya M, Morita T, Agar M, Choi YS, Goh C, et al. Palliative care development in the Asia-Pacific region: An International Survey from the Asia Pacific Hospice Palliative Care Network (APHN). BMJ Supportive & Palliative Care. 2017;**7**(1):23-31

[13] Hui D, Mori M, Watanabe SM, Caraceni A, Strasser F, Saarto T, et al. Referral criteria for outpatient specialty palliative cancer care: An international consensus. The Lancet Oncology. 2016;**17**(12):e552-e559

[14] Rassouli M, Sajjadi M. Palliative care in the Islamic Republic of Iran. In: Silberman M, editor. Palliative Care to the Cancer Patient: The Middle East as

a Model for Emerging Countries. New York: Nova; 2014

[15] Connor SR, Centeno C, Garralda E, Clelland D, Clark D. Estimating the number of patients receiving specialized palliative care globally in 2017. Journal of Pain and Symptom Management. 2021;**61**(4):812-816

[16] Reis A, Pedrosa A, Dourado M, Reis C. Information and communication technologies in long-term and palliative care. Procedia Technology. 2013;**9**:1303-1312

[17] Homsi J, Walsh D, Rivera N, Rybicki LA, Nelson KA, LeGrand SB, et al. Symptom evaluation in palliative medicine: Patient report vs systematic assessment. Supportive Care in Cancer. 2006;**14**(5):444-453

[18] Currow DC, Allingham S, Yates P, Johnson C, Clark K, Eagar K. Improving national hospice/palliative care service symptom outcomes systematically through point-of-care data collection, structured feedback and benchmarking. Supportive Care in Cancer. 2015;**23**(2): 307-315

[19] Haun MW, Estel S, Rücker G, Friederich HC, Villalobos M, Thomas M, et al. Early palliative care for adults with advanced cancer. Cochrane Database of Systematic Reviews. 2017;**12**(6):6

[20] Clark D. Total pain', disciplinary power and the body in the work of Cicely Saunders, 1958-1967. Social Science & Medicine. 1999;**49**(6):727-736

[21] Al Saraireh FA, Aloush SM, Al Azzam M, Al Bashtawy M. The effectiveness of cognitive behavioral therapy versus psychoeducation in the management of depression among patients undergoing haemodialysis. Issues in Mental Health Nursing. 2018;**39**(6):514-518

[22] Karim SM, Zekri J, Abdelghany E, Dada R, Munsoor H, Ahmad I. Time from last chemotherapy to death and its correlation with the end of life care in a referral hospital. Indian Journal of Medical and Paediatric Oncology. 2015;**36**(1):55

[23] Pritchard S, Cuvelier G, Harlos M, Barr R. Palliative care in adolescents and young adults with cancer. Cancer. 2011;**117**(S10):2323-2328

[24] Temel JS, Greer JA, El-Jawahri A, Pirl WF, Park ER, Jackson VA, et al. Effects of early integratedpalliative care in patients with lung and GI cancer: A randomized clinical trial. Journal of Clinical Oncology. 2017;**35**(8):834

[25] Ferrell BR, Temel JS, Temin S, Smith TJ. Integration of palliative care into standard oncology care: ASCO clinical practice guideline update summary. Journal of Oncology Practice/ American Society of Clinical Oncology. 2017;**13**(2):119-121

[26] Hui D et al. Concepts and definitions for "supportive care," "best supportive care," "palliative care," and "hospice care" in the published literature, dictionaries, and textbooks. Supportive Care in Cancer. 2013;**21**(3):659-685

[27] Smith TH, Cassel JB. Cost and non-clinical outcomes of palliative care. Journal of Pain and Symptom Management. 2009;**38**:32-44

[28] Goodarzi E, Sohrabivafa M, Adineh HA, Moayed L, Khazaei Z. Geographical distribution global incidence and mortality of lung cancer and its relationship with the Human Development Index (HDI); an ecology

study in 2018. World Cancer Research Journal. 2019;**6**:11

[29] Goldstraw P, Chansky K, Crowley J, Rami-Porta R, Asamura H, Eberhardt WE, et al. The IASLC lung cancer staging project: Proposals for revision of the TNM stage groupings in the forthcoming (eighth) edition of the TNM classification for lung cancer. Journal of Thoracic Oncology: Official Publication of the International Association for the Study of Lung Cancer. 2016;**11**(1):39-51

[30] Wao H, Mhaskar R, Kumar A, Miladinovic B, Djulbegovic B. Survival of patients with non-small cell lung cancer without treatment: A systematic review and meta-analysis. Systematic Reviews. 2013;**2**:10

[31] Iyer S, Roughley A, Rider A, Taylor-Stokes G. The symptom burden of non-small cell lung cancer in the USA: A real-world crosssectional study. Supportive Care in Cancer. 2014;**22**(1):181-187

[32] NCCN Guidelines® for Palliative Care Version 1. 2018. Available from: https://www.nccn.org/professionals/physician_gls/pdf/palliative.pdf [Accessed: April 2018]

[33] Shih A, Jackson KC 2nd. Role of corticosteroids in palliative care. Journal of Pain & Palliative Care Pharmacotherapy. 2007;**21**(4):69-76

[34] Lossignol D. A little help from steroids in oncology. Journal of Translational Internal Medicine. 2016;**4**(1):52-54

[35] Masuda E, Sista AK, Pua BB, Madoff DC. Palliative procedures in lung cancer. Seminars in Interventional Radiology. 2013;**30**(2):199-205

[36] Farbicka P, Nowicki A. Palliative care in patients with lung cancer. Contemporary Oncology. 2013;**17**(3):238-245

[37] Jassem E, Batura-Gabryel H, Cofta S, et al. Reccomendation of Polish Respiratory Society for palliative care in chronic lung diseases. Pulmonology and Allergology. 2012;**80**:41-64

[38] Jassem E, Jassem J. Duszność w przebiegu raka płuca. Polish Medical. 2002;**1**:3-10

[39] Kloke M, Cherny N. Treatment of dyspnoea in advanced cancer patients: ESMO Clinical Practice Guidelines. Annals of Oncology. 2015;**26**:v169-v173

[40] Navigante AH, Cerchietti LC, Castro MA, Lutteral MA, Cabalar ME. Midazolam as adjunct therapy tomorphine in the alleviation of severe dyspnea perception in patients with advanced cancer. Journal of Pain and Symptom Management. 2006;**31**(1):38-47

[41] Wildiers H, Dhaenekint C, Demeulenaere P, Clement PM, Desmet M, Van Nuffelen R, et al. Atropine, hyoscine butylbromide, or scopolamine are equally effective for the treatment of death rattle in terminal care. Journal of Pain and Symptom Management. 2009;**38**(1):124-133

[42] Back IN, Jenkins K, Blower A, Beckhelling J. A study comparing hyoscine hydrobromide and glycopyrrolate in the treatment of death rattle. Palliative Medicine. 2001;**15**(4):329-336

[43] Leppert W. Leczenie objawów ze strony układu oddechowego u chorych na nowotwory. Nowiny Lekarskie. 2011;**80**:32-46

[44] Ferrel B, Levy MH, Paice J. Managing pain from advanced cancer in the palliative care setting. Clinical Journal of Oncology Nursing. 2008;**12**:575-581

[45] Molassiotis A, Smith JA, Bennett MI, Blackhall F, Taylor D, Zavery B, et al. Clinical expert guidelines for the management of cough in lung cancer: Report of a UK task group on cough. Cough. 2010;**6**:9

[46] Warren P, Burke C. Endovascular management of chronic upper extremity deep vein thrombosis and superior vena cava syndrome. Seminars in Interventional Radiology. 2011;**28**: 32-38

[47] Mucke M, Mochamat, Cuhls H, Peuckmann-Post V, Minton O, Stone P, et al. Pharmacological treatments for fatigue associated with palliative care: Executive summary of a cochrane collaboration systematic review. Journal of Cachexia, Sarcopenia and Muscle. 2016;**7**(1):23-27

[48] Cramp F, Byron-Daniel J. Exercise for the management of cancer-related fatigue in adults. Cochrane Database of Systematic Reviews. 2012;**11**:11

[49] Dionne-Odom JN, Hull JG, Martin MY, Lyons KD, Prescott AT, Tosteson T, et al. Associations between advanced cancer patients' survival and family caregiver presence and burden. Cancer Medicine. 2016;**5**(5):853-862

[50] Martin VR. Ovarian cancer. In: Henke YC, Wujcik D, Gobel BH, editors. Cancer Nursing Principles and Practice. 7th ed. 2011. pp. 1546-1579

[51] Mirza MR, Coleman RL, González-Martín A, Moore KN, Colombo N, Ray-Coquard I, et al. The forefront of ovarian cancer therapy: Update on PARP inhibitors. Annals of Oncology. 2020;**31**(9):1148-1159

[52] Tew WP, Lacchetti C, Ellis A, Maxian K, Banerjee S, Bookman M, et al. PARP inhibitors in the management of ovarian cancer: ASCO guideline. Obstetrical & Gynecological Survey. 2020;**75**(12):739-741

[53] Mendiola C, Valdiviezo N, Vega E, Sanchez Munoz A, Ciruelos EM, Manso L, et al. Altretamine for recurrent ovarian cancer or as maintenance after response to second-line therapy. Journal of Clinical Oncology. 2011;**29**(15_suppl):e15589

[54] Talwar V, Goel V, Raina S, Patnaik N, Doval DC. Altretamine in advanced pretreated epithelial ovarian carcinoma patients: Experience from a center in North India. Current Medicine Research and Practice. 2016;**6**(3):109-112

[55] Cannistra SA, Gershenson DM, Recht A. Ovarian Cancer, Fallopian Tube Carcinoma, and Peritoneal Carcinoma. Cancer: Principles and Practise of Oncology. 9th ed. Philadelphia: Lippincott Williams & Wilkins; 2011. pp. 1368-1391

[56] Morgan M, Boyd J, Drapkin R, Seiden MV. Ch 89—Cancers arising in the ovary. In: Clinical Oncology. 5th ed. Philadelphia, PA: Elsevier; 2014. p. 1592

[57] Target Ovarian Cancer. Controlling Your Symptoms. 2017. Available from: https://targetovariancancer.org.uk/information-and-support/my-ovarian-cancer-incurable/controlling-your-symptoms

[58] Mayo Clinic Staff. Ovarian Cancer. 2018. Available from: https://mayoclinic.org/diseases-conditions/ovarian-cancer/basics/definition/con-20028096

[59] Peng X, et al. Randomized clinical trial comparing octreotide and scopolamine butylbromide in symptom control of patients with inoperable bowel obstruction due to advanced ovarian cancer. 2015;**13**(1):1-6

[60] Treating Ovarian Cancer. n.d. Available from: https://cancer.org/cancer/ovariancancer/detailedguide/ovarian-cancer-treating-general-info

[61] What is Ovarian Cancer? 2018. Available from: https://cancer.org/cancer/ovariancancer/detailedguide/ovarian-cancer-what-is-ovarian-cancer

[62] Hernandez RK, Wade SW, Reich A, Pirolli M, Liede A, Lyman GH. Incidence of bone metastases in patients with solid tumors: Analysis of oncology electronic medical records in the United States. BMC Cancer. 2018;**18**(1):1-1

[63] Heindel W, Gübitz R, Vieth V, Weckesser M, Schober O, Schäfers M. The diagnostic imaging of bone metastases. Deutsches Ärzteblatt International. 2014;**111**(44):741

[64] Handkiewicz-Junak D, Poeppel TD, Bodei L, Aktolun C, Ezziddin S, Giammarile F, et al. EANM guidelines for radionuclide therapy of bone metastases with beta-emitting radionuclides. European Journal of Nuclear Medicine and Molecular Imaging. 2018;**45**:846-859

[65] Michael H-H, Tsai Y-Y, Ho_e, S.E. Overview of diagnosis and management of metastatic disease to bone. Cancer Control. 2012;**19**:84-91

[66] Mercadante S. Malignant bone pain: Pathophysiology and treatment. Pain. 1997;**69**:1-18

[67] Roodman GD. Mechanisms of bone metastasis. The New England Journal of Medicine. 2004;**350**(16):1655-1664

[68] Yoneda T, Hiasa M, Nagata Y, Okui T, White FA. Acidic microenvironment and bone pain in cancer-colonized bone. BoneKEy Reports. 2015;**4**. p. 690

[69] Mantyh P. Bone cancer pain: Causes, consequences, and therapeutic opportunities. Pain. 2013;**154**:54-62

[70] Zajączkowska R, Kocot-Kępska M, Leppert W, Wordliczek J. Bone pain in cancer patients: Mechanisms and current treatment. International Journal of Molecular Sciences. 2019;**20**(23):6047

[71] Iqbal MS, Kelly C, Kovarik J, Goranov B, Shaikh G, Morgan D, et al. Palliative radiotherapy for locally advanced non-metastatic head and neck cancer: A systematic review. Radiotherapy and Oncology. 2018;**126**(3):558-567

[72] Barker HE, Paget JT, Khan AA, Harrington KJ. The tumour microenvironment after radiotherapy: Mechanisms of resistance and recurrence. Nature Reviews. Cancer. 2015;**15**(7):409-425

[73] Vermorken JB, Mesia R, Rivera F, Remenar E, Kawecki A, Rottey S, et al. Platinum-based chemotherapy plus cetuximab in head and neck cancer. The New England Journal of Medicine. 2008;**359**(11):1116-1127

[74] Vermorken JB, Remenar E, Van Herpen C, Gorlia T, Mesia R, Degardin M, et al. Cisplatin, fluorouracil, and docetaxel in unresectable head and neck cancer. The New England Journal of Medicine. 2007;**357**(17):1695-1704

[75] Saito AM, Landrum MB, Neville BA, Ayanian JZ, Earle CC. The effect on survival of continuing chemotherapy to near death. BMC Palliative Care. 2011;**10**(1):1-1

[76] Caponigro F, Massa E, Manzione L, Rosati G, Biglietto M, De Lucia L, et al. Docetaxel and cisplatin in locally advanced or metastatic squamous-cell carcinoma of the head and neck: A phase II study of the Southern Italy Cooperative Oncology Group (SICOG). Annals of Oncology. 2001;**12**(2):199-202

[77] Manafi-Farid R, Masoumi F, Divband G, Saidi B, Ataeinia B, Hertel F, et al. Targeted palliative radionuclide therapy for metastatic bone pain. Journal of Clinical Medicine. 2020;**9**(8):2622

[78] Yadav D, Lowenfels AB. The epidemiology of pancreatitis and pancreatic cancer. Gastroenterology. 2013;**144**(6):1252-1261

[79] Bray F, Ferlay J, Soerjomataram I, Siegel RL, Torre LA, Jemal A. Global cancer statistics 2018: GLOBOCAN estimates of incidence and mortality worldwide for 36 cancers in 185 countries. CA: A Cancer Journal for Clinicians. 2018;**68**(6):394-424

[80] Maisonneuve P, Lowenfels AB. Epidemiology of pancreatic cancer: An update. Digestive Diseases. 2010;**28**(4-5):645-656

[81] Kanno A, Masamune A, Hanada K, Kikuyama M, Kitano M. Advances in early detection of pancreatic cancer. Diagnostics. 2019;**9**(1). p. 18

[82] Betés M, González Vázquez S, Bojórquez A, Lozano MD, Echeveste JI, García Albarrán L, et al. Metastatic tumors in the pancreas: The role of endoscopic ultrasound-guided fine-needle aspiration. Revista Española de Enfermedades Digestivas. 2019;**111**(5):345-350

[83] De Luca L, Repici A, Koçollari A, Auriemma F, Bianchetti M, Mangiavillano B. Pancreatoscopy: An update. World Journal of Gastrointestinal Endoscopy. 2019;**11**(1):22-30

[84] Winter JM, Brennan MF, Tang LH, et al. Survival after resection of pancreatic adenocarcinoma: Results from a single institution over three decades. Annals of Surgical Oncology. 2012;**19**(1):169-175

[85] Konstantinidis IT, Warshaw AL, Allen JN, et al. Pancreatic ductal adenocarcinoma: Is there a survival difference for R1 resections versus locally advanced unresectable tumors? What is a "true" R0 resection? Annals of Surgery. 2013;**257**(4):731-736

[86] Stathis A, Moore MJ. Advanced pancreatic carcinoma: Current treatment and future challenges. Nature Reviews. Clinical Oncology. 2010;**7**(3):163-172

[87] Dimou F, Sineshaw H, Parmar AD, Tamirisa NP, Jemal A, Riall TS. Trends in receipt and timing of multimodality therapy in early-stage pancreatic cancer. Journal of Gastrointestinal Surgery. 2016;**20**(1):93-103

[88] Evans DB, Varadhachary GR, Crane CH, et al. Preoperative gemcitabine-based chemoradiation for patients with resectable adenocarcinoma of the pancreatic head. Journal of Clinical Oncology. 2008;**26**(21):3496-3502

[89] Varadhachary GR, Wolff RA, Crane CH, et al. Preoperative gemcitabine and cisplatin followed by gemcitabine-based chemoradiation for resectable adenocarcinoma of the pancreatic head. Journal of Clinical Oncology. 2008;**26**(21):3487-3495

[90] Christians KK, Heimler JW, George B, et al. Survival of patients with resectable pancreatic cancer who received neoadjuvant therapy. Surgery. 2016;**159**(3):893-900

[91] Stark A, Hines OJ. Endoscopic and operative palliation strategies for pancreatic ductal adenocarcinoma. Seminars in Oncology. 2015;**42**(1):163-176

[92] House MG, Choti MA. Palliative therapy for pancreatic/biliary cancer. The Surgical Clinics of North America. 2005;**85**(2):359-371

[93] Maire F, Sauvanet A. Palliation of biliary and duodenal obstruction in patients with unresectable pancreatic cancer: Endoscopy or surgery? Journal of Visceral Surgery. 2013;**150**(3):S27-S31

[94] Lillemoe KD, Cameron JL, Hardacre JM, et al. Is prophylactic gastrojejunostomy indicated for unresectable periampullary cancer? A prospective randomized trial. Annals of Surgery. 1999;**230**(3):322-328

[95] Van Heek NT, DeCastro SM, van Eijck CH, et al. The need for a prophylactic gastrojejunostomy for unresectable periampullary cancer: A prospective randomized multicenter trial with special focus on assessment of quality of life. Annals of Surgery. 2003;**238**(6):894-902

[96] Gurusamy KS, Kumar S, Davidson BR. Prophylactic gastrojejunostomy for unresectable periampullary carcinoma. Cochrane Database of Systematic Reviews. 2013;**2**

[97] Dallos MC, Eisenberger AB, Bates SE. Prevention of venous thromboembolism in pancreatic cancer: Breaking down a complex clinical dilemma. The Oncologist. 2020;**25**(2):132-139

[98] Jensen SB, Pedersen AM, Vissink A, Andersen E, Brown CG, Davies AN, et al. A systematic review of salivary gland hypofunction and xerostomia induced by cancer therapies: Prevalence, severity and impact on quality of life. Supportive Care in Cancer. 2010;**18**(8):1039-1060

[99] Pedersen AM, Bardow A, Jensen SB, Nauntofte B. Saliva and gastrointestinal functions of taste, mastication, swallowing and digestion. Oral Diseases. 2002;**8**(3):117-129

[100] Toth BB, Chambers MS, Fleming TJ, Lemon JC, Martin JW. Minimizing oral complications of cancer treatment. Oncology (Williston Park, N.Y.). 1995;**9**(9):851

[101] Toth BB, Chambers MS, Fleming TC. Prevention and management of oral complications associated with cancer therapies: Radiotherapy/chemotherapy. Texas Dental Journal. 1996;**113**(6):23-29

[102] Oneschuk D, Hanson J, Bruera E. A survey of mouth pain and dryness in patients with advanced cancer. Supportive Care in Cancer. 2000;**8**(5):372-376

[103] Sweeney MP, Bagg J, Baxter WP, Aitchison TC. Oral disease in terminally ill cancer patients with xerostomia. Oral Oncology. 1998;**34**(2):123-126

[104] Öhrn KE, Wahlin YB, Sjödén PO. Oral status during radiotherapy and chemotherapy: A descriptive study of patient experiences and the occurrence of oral complications. Supportive Care in Cancer. 2001;**9**(4):247-257

[105] Hammerlid E, Mercke C, Sullivan M, Westin T. A prospective quality of life study of patients with oral or pharyngeal carcinoma treated with external beam irradiation with or without brachytherapy. Oral Oncology. 1997;**33**(3):189-196

[106] Takahashi Y. Influences of oral health-related quality of life of cancer

patients in the terminal phase. Journal of the Japanese Society for Disability and Oral Health. 2011;**5**:23-37

[107] Davies A, Finlay I. Oral care in advanced disease. Oral Care in Advanced Disease. 2011:1-250

[108] Sweeney MP, Bagg J. The mouth and palliative care. The American Journal of Hospice & Palliative Care. 2000;**17**(2):118-124

[109] Treister NS, Villa DA, Thompson L. Palliative care: Overview of mouth care at the end of life. Depression. 2020;**3**:7

[110] Wu TY, Liu HY, Wu CY, Chen HC, Huang ST, Chen PH. Professional oral care in end-of-life patients with advanced cancers in a hospice ward: Improvement of oral conditions. BMC Palliative Care. 2020;**19**(1):1-5

[111] Mehra R, Cohen RB, Burtness BA. The role of cetuximab for the treatment of squamous cell carcinoma of the head and neck. Clinical Advances in Hematology & Oncology. 2008;**6**(10):742-750

[112] Floriano TF, Heguedusch D, Pareja GN, Oliveira SV, Domaneschi C, de Barros Gallo C. Dental management in palliative care of a patient with advanced oral cancer: A case report. Journal of Oral Diagnosis. 2021;**6**(1):1-6

[113] McDermott JD, Eguchi M, Stokes WA, Amini A, Hararah M, Ding D, et al. Short-and long-term opioid use in patients with oral and oropharynx cancer. Otolaryngology – Head and Neck Surgery. 2019;**160**(3):409-419

[114] Sekido K, Tomihara K, Horikawa H, Tachinami H, Murakami N, Noguchi M. Successful control of opioid-refractory cancer pain with methadone in a patient with advanced oral squamous cell carcinoma: A case report. Oral Science International. 2018;**15**(2):78-80

[115] Elad S, Horowitz R, Zadik Y. Supportive and Palliative Care in Dentistry and Oral Medicine. The Art and Science of Palliative Medicine. Hong Kong: AME Publishing Company; 2014. pp. 385-405

[116] Arjan V et al. Clinical management of salivary gland hypofunction and xerostomia in head-and-neck cancer patients: Snccesses and barriers. International Journal of Radiation Oncology, Biology, Physics. 2010;**78**(4):983-991

[117] Jham BC, Teixeira IV, Aboud CG, Carvalho AL, Coelho Mde M, et al. A randomized phase III prospective trial of bethanechol to prevent radiotherapy-induced salivary gland damage in patients with head and neck cancer. Oral Oncology. 2007;**43**:137-142

[118] Jaguar GC, Lima EN, Kowalski LP, Pellizzon AC, Carvalho AL, et al. Double blind randomized prospective trial of bethanechol in the prevention of radiation-induced salivary gland dysfunction in head and neck cancer patients. Radiotherapy and Oncology. 2015;**115**:253-256

[119] Park B, Noh H, Choi DJ. Herbal medicine for xerostomia in cancer patients: A systematic review of randomized controlled trials. Integrative Cancer Therapies. 2018;**17**(2):179-191

[120] Ni X, Yu Y, Tian T, Liu L, Li X, Li F, et al. Acupuncture for patients with cancer-induced xerostomia: A systematic review protocol. BMJ Open. 2019;**9**(12):e031892

[121] Berk LB, Shivnani AT, Small W Jr. Pathophysiology and management of radiation-induced xerostomia.

The Journal of Supportive Oncology. 2005;**3**:191-200

[122] Coppes RP, Zeilstra LJW, Kapinga HH, Konings AWT. Early to late sparing of radiation damage to the parotid gland by adrenergic and muscarinic receptor agonists. British Journal of Cancer. 2001;**85**:1055-1063

[123] Ravasco P. Aspects of taste and compliance in patients with cancer. European Journal of Oncology Nursing. 2005;**9**:S84-S91

[124] Afraseyabi S, Afkhamzadeh A, Sabori H, Verdi F, Khaksar N, Mosavei B. Oral candidiasis amongst cancer patients at Qods Hospitals in Sanandaj. African Journal of Clinical and Experimental Microbiology. 2011;**12**(3):1595-1689

[125] Lalla RV, Latortue MC, Hong CH, et al. A systematic review of oral fungal infections in patients receiving cancer therapy. Supportive Care in Cancer. 2010;**18**(8):985-992

[126] Brondel L, Jacquin A, Meillon S, Pénicaud L. Le goût: Physiologie, rôles et dysfonctionnements. Nutrition Clinique et Métabolisme. 2013;**27**(3):123-133

[127] Malaty J, Malaty IA. Smell and taste disorders in primary care. American Family Physician. 2013;**88**(12):852-859

[128] Halyard MY, Jatoi A, Sloan JA, Bearden JD III, Vora SA, Atherton PJ, et al. Does zinc sulfate prevent therapy-induced taste alterations in head and neck cancer patients? Results of phase III double-blind, placebo-controlled trial from the North Central Cancer Treatment Group (N01C4). International Journal of Radiation Oncology, Biology, Physics. 2007;**67**(5):1318-1322

[129] Mizukami Y, Sato J, Nihei S, Kashiwaba M, Kudo K, Okuyama H, et al. The effectiveness of polaprezinc preparation for taste alteration in cancer chemotherapy. Gan to Kagaku Ryoho. Cancer & Chemotherapy. 2016;**43**(8):979-983

[130] Kouvaris JR, Kouloulias VE, Vlahos LJ. Amifostine: The first selective-target and broad-spectrum radioprotector. The Oncologist. 2007;**12**(6):738-747

[131] Shokohi T, Bandalizadeh Z, Hedayati MT, Mayahi S. In vitro antifungal susceptibility of *Candida* species isolated from oropharyngeal lesions of patients with cancer to some antifungal agents. Jundishapur Journal of Microbiology. 2011;**4**(1):S19-S26

[132] Wl W. Scarborough je osteoradionecrosis in intra-oral cancer. American Journal of Roentgenology. 1938;**40**:524-534

[133] Silvestre-Rangil J, Silvest F-J. Clinico-theraper-rtic management of osteoradionecrosis: A literature review and update. Medicina Oral, Patología Oral y Cirugía Bucal. 2011;**16**(7):E900-E904

[134] Re M. A new concept in treatment of osteoradionecrosis. Journal of Oral and Maxillofacial Surgery. 1983;**41**:351-357

[135] Adam SJ et al. Paradigm shifts ln the management of osteoradionecrosis of mandible. Oral Oncology. 2010;**46**:95-801

[136] Roila F, Molassiotis A, Herrstedt J, Aapro M, Gralla RJ, Bruera E, et al. 2016 MASCC and ESMO guideline update for the prevention of chemotherapy- and radiotherapy-induced nausea and vomiting and of nausea and vomiting in advanced cancer patients. Annals of Oncology. 2016;**27**:v119-v133

[137] Louie KS, Mehanna H, Sasieni P. Trends in head and neck cancers in England from 1995-2011 and projections up to 2025. Oral Oncology. 2015;**51**(4):341-348

[138] Siegel RL, Miller KD, Jemal A. Cancer statistics 2017. CA: A Cancer Journal for Clinicians. 2017;**67**(1):7-30

[139] De La Cruz M, Fan J, Yennu S, Tanco K, Shin S, Wu J, et al. The frequency of missed delirium in patients referred to palliative care in a comprehensive cancer center. Supportive Care in Cancer. 2015;**23**:2427-2433

[140] Hui D. Delirium in the palliative care setting: "Sorting" out the confusion. Palliative Medicine. 2019;**33**:863-864

[141] Rudolph JL, Archambault E, Kelly B, Force VABDT. A delirium risk modification program is associated with hospitaloutcomes. Journal of the American Medical Directors Association. 2014;**15**(957):e7-e11

[142] Schoen MW, Cull S, Buckhold FR. False bed alarms: A teachable moment. JAMA Internal Medicine. 2016;**176**:741-742

[143] Grassi L, Caraceni A, Mitchell A, Nanni MG, Berardi MA, Caruso R, et al. Management of delirium in palliativecare: A review. Current Psychiatry Reports. 2015;**17**:1-9

[144] Agar MR, Lawlor PG, Quinn S, Draper B, Caplan GA, Rowett D, et al. Efficacy of oral risperidone, haloperidol, or placebo for symptoms of delirium among patients in palliative care: A randomized clinical trial. JAMA Internal Medicine. 2017;**177**:34-42

[145] Mattiuzzi C, Sanchis-Gomar F, Lippi G. Concise update on colorectal cancer epidemiology. Annals of Translational Medicine. 2019;**7**(21):609-613

[146] Rudler M et al. Optimal management of ascites. Liver International. 2020;**40**:128-135

[147] Torre LA, Bray F, Siegel RL, Ferlay J, Lortet-Tieulent J, Jemal A. Global cancer statistics, 2012. CA: A Cancer Journal for Clinicians. 2015;**65**(2):87-108

[148] National Institutes of Health National Cancer Institute. Surveillance, Epidemiology, and End Results Program. SEER Cancer Stat Facts: Bladder Cancer. Available from: https://seer.cancer.gov/statfacts/html/urinb.html [Accessed: 11 August 2017]

[149] Didkowska J, Wojciechowska U, Zatoński W. Nowotwory złośliwe w Polsce w 2011 roku. Warszawa: Krajowy Rejestr Nowotworów; 2013

[150] Oya H, Koike M, Iwata N, Kobayashi D, Matoba M. Pain management for urological cancer patients in palliative care. Journal of Palliative Care and Medicine. 2013;**3**(168):2

[151] National Collaborating Centre for Cancer (UK). Bladder Cancer: Diagnosis and Management. London: National Institute for Health and Care Excellence (NICE); 2015

[152] Suzuki K, Hanashima F, Shirotake S, Kodaira K, Nishimoto K, Takahashi T, et al. Determining the optimum way to maintain quality of life for very elderly patients with advanced bladder cancer and poor performance status: A case report. Molecular and Clinical Oncology. 2017;**6**(6):968-970

[153] Daniels CJ, Wakefield PJ, Bub GA. Bladder metastasis presenting as neck, arm and thorax pain: A case report.

Chiropractic & Manual Therapies. 2016;**24**:14

[154] Mariotto AB, Etzioni R, Hurlbert M, Penberthy L, Mayer M. Estimation of the number of women living with metastatic breast cancer in the United States. Cancer Epidemiology, Biomarkers & Prevention. 2017;**26**(6):809-815

[155] Thrift-Perry M, Cabanes A, Cardoso F, Hunt KM, Cruz TA, Faircloth K. Global analysis of metastatic breast cancer policy gaps and advocacy efforts across the patient journey. Breast. 2018;**41**:93-106

[156] Dange VN, Shid SJ, Magdum CS, Mohite SK. A review on breast cancer: An overview. Asian Journal of Pharmaceutical Research. 2017;**7**(1):49-51

[157] Hariramani N, Jayanthi S. A systematic review of intrinsic factors and its influence in breast cancer. Research Journal of Pharmacy and Technology. 2018;**11**(8):3543-3546

[158] Jayashree V, Velraj M. Breast cancer and various prognostic biomarkers for the diagnosis of the disease: A review. Research Journal of Pharmacy and Technology. 2017;**10**(9):3211-3216

[159] Yadav AR, Mohite SK. Cancer—A silent killer: An overview. Asian Journal of Pharmaceutical Research. 2020;**10**(3):213-216

[160] Cleeland CS, Gonin R, Hatfield AK, et al. Pain and its treatment in outpatients with metastatic cancer. The New England Journal of Medicine. 1994;**330**:592-596

[161] Li BT, Wong MH, Pavlakis N. Treatment and prevention of bone metastases from breast cancer: A comprehensive review of evidence for clinical practice. Journal of Clinical Medicine. 2014;**3**(1):1-24

[162] Mercadante S, Fulfaro F. Management of painful bone metastases. Current Opinion in Oncology. 2007;**19**(4):308-314

[163] Ripamonti CL, Santini D, Maranzano E, Berti M, Roila F. ESMO Guidelines Working Group. Management of cancer pain: ESMO clinical practice guidelines. Annals of Oncology. 2012;**23**:vii139-vii154

[164] Cherny NI, Paluch-Shimon S, Berner-Wygoda Y. Palliative care: Needs of advanced breast cancer patients. Breast Cancer: Targets and Therapy. 2018;**10**:231

[165] Juvet LK, Thune I, Elvsaas IKØ, et al. The effect of exercise on fatigue and physical functioning in breast cancer patients during and after treatment and at 6-month follow-up: A meta-analysis. Breast. 2017;**33**:166-177

[166] Mohandas H, Jaganathan SK, Mani MP, Ayyar M, Rohini Thevi GV. Cancer-related fatigue treatment: An overview. Journal of Cancer Research and Therapeutics. 2017;**13**(6):916-929

[167] Brunault P, Champagne AL, Huguet G. Major depressive disorder, personality disorders, and coping strategies are independent risk factors for lower quality of life in non-metastatic breast cancer patients. Psycho-Oncology. 2016;**25**:513-520

[168] Park EM, Gelber S, Rosenberg SM, et al. Anxiety and depression in young women with metastatic breast cancer: A cross-sectional study. Psychosomatics. 2018;**59**(3):251-258

[169] Rodin G. Effective treatment for depression in patients with cancer. Lancet. 2014;**384**(9948):1076-1078

[170] Li M, Kennedy EB, Byrne N, Gerin-Lajoie C, Green E, Katz MR, et al. The Management of Depression in Patients with Cancer. Vol. 11. Toronto: Cancer Care Ontario; 2015. pp. 19-14

[171] Łuczak J, Kotlińska-Lemieszek A. Opieka paliatywna/hospicyjna/ medycyna paliatywna. Nowiny Lekarskie. 2011;**80**:3-15

Chapter 9

Feeding at the End of Life in Brazilian Amazon: Qualitative Analysis of Medical Indications

Caroline Anjos, Katherine Dambrowski, Antonio Godoy and Paula Barrioso

Abstract

Background: Death is preceded by several medical decisions that impact the dying process. One of the challenges faced by the multidisciplinary team regarding the care for patients at the end of life process is the indication or interruption of enteral feeding. The aim of this study was to describe the decision experience of the indication of artificial nutrition for seriously ill patients at the end of life by physicians working in a private oncology clinic in Manaus-Amazonas (AM), and their perceptions about end-of-life process. Material and Methods: A cross-sectional and observational study based on a qualitative approach. A clinical case involving a hypothetical patient with advanced dementia, not a candidate for disease-modifying therapy, evolving with signs of end of life was applied. The doctors answered in a discursive manner a question about which nutritional option would be the most adequate. Content analysis was used to analyze the data. Results: A total number of 15 specialists physicians acting in a private oncologic clinic in Manaus-AMwere included. Approximately 42.84% of respondents opted to indicate the placement of a nasoenteric feeding tube or a gastrostomy. A large portion of them believed that the patient had the opportunity to treat severe dementia. Conclusions: There is little scientific evidence of the benefits of using artificial feeding in elderly patients with advanced dementia. Further studies are needed in addition to continuing educating initiatives to inform prescribing professionals about the potential related risks of artificial diet at the end of life.

Keywords: palliative care, death, diet, Brazil, elderly

1. Introduction

Death is preceded by several medical decisions that directly impact how the dying process will happen [1]. Despite being a sensitive topic for many professionals, being able to make proportional decisions has a significant weight in the last days of life [2]. The process to decide should be a common practice among physicians, especially when they care for patients with advanced diseases. However, many of them still face problems associated with indications or interruption of treatments during the trajectory of some illnesses [3].

All life-limiting diseases have specificities during the final phase of life, some are better defined, such as cancer and others as dementia could be more complex to manage. The survival rate for dementia is around 3 to 10 years. Dementia has a trajectory with progressive losses and decreasing performance that can persist for years [4, 5]. An important dilemma for all progressive conditions is about feeding in the last days of life. The patient in the dying process reduces food intake, progressing in most cases to complete fasting. However, both the medical team and the family question the lack of food offered in this stage of disease evolution [6].

Evidence-based guidelines and approaches that incorporate quality of life and patient preferences as Palliative Care (PC) may help solve this problem [7]. Palliative Care is a holistic approach that aims to alleviate the suffering caused by serious and progressive illnesses. The goal is to maintain the highest possible quality of life in the face of these conditions. It is a person-centered approach where the object of care is the patient, family, and caregivers. In general, provides skills for decision-makers concerning end-of-life dilemmas and affords tools to align care trajectory with patient values and preferences [8].

The incorporation of PC approach in the standard care improves the decision-making process, the symptoms control in the last moments of life, and improve communication with the family [9]. However, the lack of education in palliative care among doctors has been one of the most common barriers in providing quality palliative care. Many studies have revealed that professionals often have inadequate knowledge of pain, the use of opioids, management symptoms, and the concept of palliative care and its indications. Public awareness and acceptance of the end of life should involve educational initiatives not only for health professionals but the entire community [10–12].

Given the above considerations, to understand how medical professionals deal with the decision for nutrition at the end of life and also to start studies related to this topic, the objective of the present investigation was to describe the decision experience of the indication of artificial nutrition for seriously ill patients at the end of life.

2. Methods

This was a cross-sectional and observational study based on a qualitative approach, which was approved by the local Ethics Committee under protocol number 2.925.747/2018. The study was carried out in the steps that follow: 1) The physicians included were approached individually and informed about the objective and methodology of the study. Those who agreed to participate signed written informed consent; 2) After that, each doctor received by e-mail, through google.docs, a clinical case involving a hypothetical patient with advanced dementia, who was not a candidate for disease-modifying therapy, admitted to the hospital with a respiratory infection secondary to bronchoaspiration, and with subsequent evolution involving end of life signs (**Table 1**); 3) Doctors had to analyzed the clinical case and then they had to answer a single question about which nutritional option would be the most suitable in that clinical situation.

Discursive responses were collected between December 2018 and March 2019 and confindentiality was guaranteed throughout the Project. The authors used the SRQR checklist when writing our report as a requirement for qualitative studies [13].

M.A.S.S., 86 years old, female, admitted in the emergency with productive cough (hyaline expectoration) and report of the caregiver of post-eating gags. The caregiver is her only child, 62 years old, no children, single, exclusive caregiver of the mother in the last 3 years when she had to abandon her job to dedicate herself to her mother exclusively.
Vital signs: PA = 90 x40mmHg; FC = 104 bpm; FR = 20irpm; SatO2 = 96% (in ambient air); TAX = 36.7°C.
In view of the hypothesis of pneumonia secondary to bronchoaspiration, hospital admission was requested. Physician that receives the patient and after initial clinical measures (oxygen therapy and nebulization) the patient stay stable.
Morbid-personal antecedents: Patient with elderly's fragility syndrome and Alzheimer's dementia for about 3 years and, for about 1 year, totally dependent on basic daily activities (bathing, clothing, transference, continence, hygiene). She has been enrolled for a year with recurrent infections (pneumonia and urinary tract infection).
Already accompanied by a multidisciplinar team of palliative care since the diagnosis of dementia. She has been attending a low oral intake and coughing after feeding for 6 mouths and 1 month ago, had been treated for pneumonia with oral antibiotic. No pain or other symptoms.
Medications on use: Donepezil 10 mg/day; Lactulose 10 ml 12/12 hours.
Significant findings on physical examination: Sarcopenia, spontaneous ocular opening but not contacting, snoring transmission on the pulmonary auscultation.
In view of the clinical case presented, in the current hospitalization, we would like to know what you would be conduct in relation to food. Would you recommend the beggining of artificial diet? Justify your answer.

Table 1.
Clinical case.

3. Participants

The study was conducted at an Oncology clinic of the private health sector in Manaus-AM. The physicians were chosen to participate if they had a specialty, clinical or surgical, and at least three years of experience in their areas.

The subjects were 15 physicians working in the following specialties: Clinical Oncology (1), Radio-Oncology (3), Mastology (3), Hematology (1), Gastroenterology (1), Head and Neck Surgery (1), Digestive Tract Surgery (1), Orthopedics (1), Geriatrics (2), and Thoracic Surgery (1). Exclusion criteria were physicians not involved in the clinical care of adult patients, specialists with less than 3 years of practical clinical activity, and physicians caring exclusively for pregnant or puerperal women, children, and patients in the intensive care unit (ICU).

4. Data analysis

The discourses obtained were analyzed by Content Analysis. This methodology proposes a set of techniques for the analysis of verbal communication to obtain indicators, qualitative or not, that will permit the description of the content of the messages of the persons interviewed. The method consists of three phases (analysis, exploration of the material and treatment of the results, inference, and interpretation) and one of the criteria for data categorization can be a semantic one or a thematic one when all topics having the same meaning are grouped. All the discourses were transcribed in their entirety.

5. Results

Among the 15 physicians included, only one did not complete the stages of the study and was excluded. They were divided in the following specialties: Clinical oncology (1); Radio-oncology (3); Mastology (3); Hematology (1); Head an neck surgery (1); Thoracic surgery (1); Digestive system surgery (1); Geriatric (2) and Orthopedic (1). The others informations about the physicians included are in **Table 2**.

Regarding the indication of an alternative nutritional route for an artificial diet at the time of hospitalization of a patient with advanced dementia and in an active dying process, the following discourses were obtained from the doctors who opted to indicate the placement of a nasoenteric feeding tube or a gastrostomy (42.84%):

"... There still is the possibility of treatment of the base disease."

"... Patient with poor performance status, functionally dependent, with aspiration pneumonia and sarcopenia. She indicates definitive enteral nutrition. I would

Variables	n (%)	Mean
Gender		
Female	5 (35.71%)	
Male	9 (64.29%)	
Age group		
25–30 years	1 (7.14%)	
31–35 years	7 (50%)	35.5 years
36–40 years	4 (28.57%)	
41–45 years	2 (14.28%)	
Marital status		
Single	4 (28.57%)	
Married	9 (64.28%)	
Divorced	1 (7.14%)	
Children		
Yes	9 (64.29%)	
No	5 (35.71%)	
Religion		
Yes	13 (92.85%)	
No	1 (7.14%)	
Specialty		
Clinical	7 (50%)	
Surgical	7 (50%)	
Practice time		
= 7 years	5 (37.71%)	
> 7 years	9 (64.28%)	

Table 2.
Social professional characteristics.

first prescribe the passage of a nasoenteric feeding tube and I would program a gastrostomy."

"... Despite the sarcopenia, the patient may still have some time of life if she responds to antibiotic therapy. If the patient does not show a satisfactory response, no invasive procedure should be indicated, and nutrition should be interrupted."

"... I would indicate enteral nutrition due to the severe status and clinical signs and symptoms of the patient."

"I would indicate endoscopic gastrostomy, which permits a satisfactory nutritional route of easy manipulation and that would avoid discomfort and frequent losses such as those occurring with nasoenteric feeding tubes."

The following responses were obtained from the professionals who were against the indication of an alternative route for an artificial diet:

"... Despite the short duration of Alzheimer's disease, the patient is in an advanced phase of the disease and is dependent on all her basic daily life activities. An alternative route (nasoenteric feeding tube or gastrostomy) is not indicated in these cases since it does not reduce the risk of aspiration. The decision is shared and, since the patient is already monitored by a PC team, probably it would be easier for her daughter to accept not to use an alternative nutrition route."

"No additional nutrition route due to the reserved clinical signs and symptoms of the patient, with no perspective of reversal of the basal clinical condition, with a strong negative impact on the quality of life of her relatives."

"... I would maintain the indication of the oral route because it would be less invasive and painful for the patient."

"... A patient with a progressive incurable disease and multiple infectious intercurrences over the last year, so that the current hospitalization could be considered to involve the end of life care."

6. Discussion

6.1 Epidemiology and dementia definition

In the US, Alzheimer's disease is a condition whose mortality has been increasing and a recent analysis has demonstrated that in 2010 about 32% of the deaths in elderly were due to the evolution and secondary complications of dementia. This number is projected to increase to 43% by 2050. According to the World Health Organization (WHO), is estimated about 50 million people with dementia around the world and is expected to triplicate this number by 2050 [14].

Several instruments have been developed to assess the severity and staging of dementias. One of these is the FAST scale (Functional Assessment Staging) and it is divided into 16 stages of progression (normal to severe dementia). FAST scale has no interference with low education and gives more details of the functional stages of severe dementia [15].

6.2 Artificial diet indication

There is little scientific evidence about the benefits of the use of artificial nutrition for older patients with advanced dementia [16, 17]. However, when feeding difficulties and weight loss occur, it is necessary to decide between about continuing to offer food by the oral route or placing a feeding tube (enteric tube or endoscopic gastrostomy) [18]. The estimate is that more than one-third of patients with severe cognitive impairment admitted on a home care basis in the US are being fed through a tube for artificial nutrition [9].

Patients with dementia usually experience feeding difficulties in addition to the decline of cognitive, language, and functional skills given the progressive neurodegenerative process. The reduction of oral intake in the presence of advanced dementia is expected, not only due to nutritional problems but also due to the natural course of the disease [18]. Another theory suggests that patients with advanced dementia have reduced calorie needs due to their low basal metabolic rate and inactivity. Besides, as is the case for other advanced clinical conditions, patients are expected to eat less as part of the natural progression towards the end of life [18, 19]. However, it is important to distinguish between death due to lack of nutrition and hydration and the dying process in which failure to eat and drink is due to the natural dying process secondary to a chronic disease in the absence of therapy that modifies the disease. In the latter case, maintaining artificial nutrition could be a form of "forced feeding" and improper treatment. However, the initiation of an artificial diet and hydration has been experienced as a basic form of care that prevents death from starvation [19].

A recent Cochrane meta-analysis concluded that the use of artificial nutrition did not prolong the survival of patients with advanced dementia compared to a comfort diet. However, most of the studies included were observational and the absence of randomized clinical studies limited the quality of information [18].

6.3 Risks of artificial diet indication

Feeding tubes are associated with countless adverse effects that have not yet been properly quantitated. The current literature suggests rates of complications ranging from 32 to 70%. Also, keeping the feeding tube properly positioned in patients with dementia it may requires physical restraint or pharmacological sedation, which may negatively affect the quality of life of patients in these conditions. The patients may also be deprived of the pleasure of eating by mouth and of the interpersonal interaction brought about by nutrition [18]. In addition, there are problems related to the inadvertent removal of the tube by the patients, leading to the need for physical or pharmacological restraint [19]. The complications most frequently described are pain and others directly related to tube placement (e.g., infection, bleeding, increased risk of aspiration, increased risk of pressure ulcers, gastrointestinal symptoms such as reflux, diarrhea and constipation, increased incidence of physical or chemical restraint to prevent tube removal by the patient, volemic overload leading to increased pulmonary edema, and peripheral edema). Also, the increase in the volume of airway secretions in the presence of edema may increase the perception of hunger [9].

When the artificial diet and hydration are discontinued, the dehydration caused is isotonic and causes less thirst than the hypertonic dehydration that occurs when only the artificial diet is discontinued. Besides, dehydration may lead to increased dying comfort because it reduces the occurrence of secretions in the respiratory and gastrointestinal systems, thus also reducing vomiting and diarrhea. It may also reduce the volume of urine in patients with incontinence, leading to fewer skin irritations. Dehydration causes a reduced release of vasopressin and there is some evidence that it also reduces the release of endorphin and the perception of pain [14].

Other mechanisms whereby the discontinuation of an artificial diet and hydration leads to more comfort for the patient, probably concerning the formation of ketone bodies. The increased formation of ketones leads also to the formation of g-aminobutyric acid which therefore acts as an inhibitory brain neurotransmitter and reduces the occurrence of convulsion [14].

6.4 Medical prescription

Physicians can prescribe artificial nutrition and hydration as a form of care based on ethical principles more than on scientific evidence and motivated by their personal belief that providing food and water satisfies basic human needs [19]. Physicians and other health professionals play an important role in the perpetuation of excessive indication and use of feeding tubes for patients with advanced dementia. One should consider some misunderstandings among these professionals, such as the fact that the risk of bronchoaspiration and pneumonia is an important factor to be considered for the indication of a feeding tube [9]. However, this scenario is not unique to Brazil. A recent systematic review shows that professionals from other countries, such as the USA, Japan and Israel, have not applied the latest evidence to their clinical practice either [20].

A systematic review of therapeutic decisions regarding artificial diet and hydration for patients at risk of reduced mental capacity has revealed that that the first reason behind the initiation of the two interventions, including patients with dementia, is to prolong life. However, there is evidence indicating that neither approach, when started in patients with advanced dementia, courses with increased survival or improves the quality of life of these patients. Indeed, enteral nutrition through a tube places the patient at risk for countless complications and deprives them of their dignity [9].

However, the absence of artificial nutrition may cause dissatisfaction among the patient's relatives since it is widely felt culturally that feeding is symbolically associated with the act of caring. Also, it is felt that, when artificial nutrition is not started, the patient will suffer hunger and thirst in the absence of adequate oral intake [18]. It is common to observe that the cultural conceptions of nutrition as "basic care" conflict with its medical-legal definition since this is a form of technological intervention. Research specifically focusing on removing or refusing nutrition and hydration has demonstrated that the ensuing death is not particularly painful. However, these investigations have been conducted only on older, frail and/or sick patients in the final phase of life [19, 21].

6.5 Recognizing signs of the end of the life

Conducting a prognostic assessment and identifying signs of an active process of death are constant challenges in medical practice. Especially between non-palliative health care professionals and the biggest difficulty to recognize signs of imminent death. The inconsistencies to make a prognostic analysis can reflect insufficient medical training in medical schools and graduate programs [22].

A recent study carried out with patients with oncological diseases in the final stage identified that for the recognition of imminent death, PPS was the most important factor among doctors, followed by the presence of Cheyne-Stokes breathing, declining clinical condition, agitation or lowering of the level of consciousness and noisy breathing due to hypersecretion of the airways in addition to peripheral cyanosis. Surprisingly, there was no difference in the ability to do prognostic analysis between older doctors, suggesting that clinical experience alone may not optimize the ability to predict [22].

Symptoms related to imminent death are: patient restricted to bed, decreased level of consciousness, patient able to swallow small sips of fluids and the patient loses the ability to ingest medications orally [23].

Both the health team and family members have doubts about the definition of end-of-life. Due to this uncertainty and the unpredictability of the evolution of the patient's condition, clinical support must be specifically focused on the individual's needs [24].

6.6 Advanced care planning

Anticipated directives were developed in the United States in the 1960s with the aim to empower patients and improve professionals' and family caregivers' compliance with patient preferences in the event of loss of decision-making capacity [25].

A recent population study has demonstrated that people are more afraid of a diagnosis of dementia than of a diagnosis of cancer (21% vs. 18%) and this fear is especially common among persons older than 60 years (29% are more afraid of being diagnosed with dementia and only 9% are more afraid of being diagnosed with cancer). There are countless reasons for this fear, among them: loss of memory, loss of autonomy, becoming dependent on another person for self-care, loss of dignity, the possibility of suffering, and the increased health costs [14].

Most insertions of a feeding tube occur during hospital admission when specialists and clinicians have no relationship with the relatives and prescribe health care under pressure from family and caregivers regarding the initiation of artificial nutrition. It is necessary to start early during the course of dementia the discussions about artificial diet and hydration [9].

Anticipated wish directives specifying whether or not the patient wishes to receive artificial nutrition and hydration if he/she should progress to an advanced stage of dementia, represent a manner of guaranteeing the autonomy of the patient, regardless of the family's desire [14].

7. Conclusion

There is little scientific evidence about the benefits of using artificial feeding among elderly patients with advanced dementia, precisely benefit of starting an artificial diet at the end of life. This is may be as a result ofthe lack of adequate medical training in this field.

Despite, medical professionals still keep using this type of health intervention in clinical practice.

Acknowledgements

This study was supported by the Clinic of Oncologic Therapy and Diagnostic Imaging (SENSUMED Oncology) and the authors had the support of an extremely competent brazilian geriatric physician: Claudia Burlá, MD.

Conflict of interest

The authors declare no conflict of interest.

DOI: http://dx.doi.org/10.5772/intechopen.104509

Funding

The authors received no financial support for the research, authorship and publication of this article.

Abbreviations

PC	Palliative care
ICU	Intensive Care Unit
WHO	World Health Organization
FAST scale	Functional Assessment Staging scale
US	United States
PPS	Palliative Performance Scale

Author details

Caroline Anjos[1], Katherine Dambrowski[2], Antonio Godoy[3]* and Paula Barrioso[4]

1 Medical Oncologist, Sensumed Oncology, Manaus, AM, Brazil

2 Medical Family and Community, Pontifical Catholic University of Paraná, Curitiba, PR, Brazil

3 Medical Oncologist, Brazil Cancer Institute, TrêsLagoas, MS, Brazil

4 Oncology and Palliative Care Nurse, Instituto Paliar, São Paulo, SP, Brazil

*Address all correspondence to: acgodoypsn@gmail.com

References

[1] Åvik Persson H, Sandgren A, Fürst C, et al. Early and late signs that precede dying among older persons in nursing homes: The multidisciplinary team's perspective. BMC Geriatrics. 2018;**18**:134. DOI: 10.1186/s12877-018-0825-0

[2] Buiting HM, Rietjens JA, Onwuteaka-Philipsen BD, van der Maas PJ, van Delden JJ, van der Heide A. A comparison of physicians' end-of-life decision making for non-western migrants and Dutch natives in the Netherlands. European Journal of Public Health. 2008;**18**:681-687 IN END OF LIFE CARE AND DECISION MAKING Opinions and experiences of the general public, bereaved relatives, and professionals

[3] Fringer A, Stangle S, Buche D, Ott SC, Schnepp W. The associations of palliative care experts regarding food refusal: A crosssectional study with an open question evaluated by triangulation analysis. PLoS One. 2020;**15**(4):e0231312. DOI: 10.1371/journal.pone.0231312

[4] van der Steen JT. Dying with dementia: What we know after more than a decade of research. Journal of Alzheimer's Disease. 2010;**22**(1):37-55

[5] Strand BH, Knapskog AB, Persson K, et al. Survival and years of life lost in various aetiologies of dementia, mild cognitive impairment (MCI) and subjective cognitive decline (SCD) in Norway. PLoS One. 2018;**13**(9):e0204436. Published 2018 Sep 21. DOI: 10.1371/journal.pone.0204436

[6] Costa MF, Soares JC. To feed and to nourish: Significances and meanings in oncologic palliative care. Revista Brasileira de Cancerologia. 2016;**62**(3):215-224

[7] Tan A, Durbin M, Chung FR, et al. Design and implementation of a clinical decision support tool for primary palliative Care for Emergency Medicine (PRIM-ER). BMC Medical Informatics Decision Making. 2020;**20**(1):13. Published 2020 Jan 28. DOI: 10.1186/s12911-020-1021-7

[8] Radbruch L, De Lima L, Knaul F, et al. Redefining palliative care-a new consensus-based definition [published online ahead of print, 2020 may 6]. Journal of Pain and Symptom Management. 2020;**S0885-3924**(20):30247-30245. DOI: 10.1016/j.jpainsymman.2020.04.027

[9] Sinuff T, Dodek P, You JJ, Barwich D, Tayler C, Downar J, et al. Improving end-of-life communication and decision making: The development of a conceptual framework and quality indicators. Journal of Pain and Symptom Management. 2015;**49**(6)

[10] Aldridge MD, Hasselar J, Garralda E, et al. Education, implementation, and policy barriers to greater integration of palliative care: A literature review. Palliative Medicine. 2016;**30**:224-239

[11] Kovásc MJ. Educação para a morte: desafionaformação de profissionais de saúde e educação. São Paulo: Casa do Psicólogo; 2003. p. 178

[12] Xie Y, Xu Y, Yang S, et al. Investigation of the awareness of and demand for hospice care and attitudes towards life-sustaining treatment at the end of life among community residents in Hangzhou. BMC Palliative Care. 2020;**19**:128. DOI: 10.1186/s12904-020-00628-8

[13] O'Brien BC, Harris IB, Beckman TJ, Reed DA, Cook DA. Standards for

reporting qualitative research: A synthesis of recommendations. Academic Medicine. 2014;**89**(9):1245-1251

[14] Vellani S. Enteral versus oral feeding in advanced dementia. Journal of the American Association of Nurse Practitioners. 2019

[15] Reisberg B. Functional assessment staging (FAST). Psychopharmacology Bulletin. 1988;**24**:653-659

[16] Volicer L, Stets K. Acceptability of an advance directive that limits food and liquids in advanced dementia. The American Journal of Hospice & Palliative Care. 2016;**33**(1):55-63

[17] Sampson E, et al, Candy B, Jones L. Enteral tube feeding for older people with advanced dementia (review). Cochrane Database of Systematic Reviews 2009, Issue 2. Art. No.: CD007209. DOI: 10.1002/14651858. CD007209.pub2.

[18] Komiya K et al. Medical professionals' attitudes toward tube feeding for themselves or their families: A multicenter survey in Japan. Journal of Palliative Medicine. 2012;**15**(5):561-566

[19] Ying I. Artificial nutrition and hydration in advanced dementia. Canadian Family Physician. 2015;**61**(3): 245-248

[20] Baumstarck K, Boyer L, Pauly V, et al. Use of artificial nutrition near the end of life: Results from a French national population-based study of hospitalized cancer patients. Cancer Medicine. 2020;**9**(2):530-540. DOI: 10.1002/cam4.2731

[21] Valentini E et al. Artificial nutrition and hydration in terminally ill patients with advanced dementia: Opinions and correlates among Italian physicians and nurses. Journal of Palliative Medicine. 2014;**17**(10):1143-1149

[22] White N et al. How do palliative care doctors recognize imminently dying patients? A judgement analysis. BMJ Open. 2018;**8**:e024996. DOI: 10.1136/ bmjopen-2018-024996

[23] Ellershaw J, Ward C. Care of the dying patient: The last hours or days of life. BMJ. 2003;**326**:30-34

[24] Browne B, Kupeli N, Moore KJ, Sampson EL, Davies N. Defining end of life in dementia: A systematic review. Palliative Medicine. 2021;**35**(10):1733-1746. DOI: 10.1177/02692163211025457

[25] Bosisio F, Sterie AC, Rubli Truchard E, Jox RJ. Implementing advance care planning in early dementia care: Results and insights from a pilot interventional trial. BMC Geriatrics. 2021;**21**(1):573. Published 2021 Oct 19. DOI: 10.1186/s12877-021-02529-8

Chapter 10

Leaving Early: The Reality of Assisted Suicide and Euthanasia in 2022

Michael H. Plumer and Margaret C. Cecil

Abstract

If cancer becomes a terminal illness, cancer patients may want to consider their options for managing the end of life. Palliative care and hospice give patients control over pain and symptoms at the end of life, but patients may want to know how to pursue more direct actions to end a life that feels too burdensome. This chapter provides a nonjudgmental look at legal ways to end one's own life in 2022. Where is assisted suicide legal in the world, including a detailed look at laws in those United States of America (USA) states that protect it? Where can a doctor provide and administer lethal drugs, providing euthanasia? What restrictions to access exist? What help and guidance are available? What options realistically exist beyond prescribed drugs, without turning to firearms and leaping from buildings? This chapter is not a how-to-end-it guide, but a brief survey of the options a patient might feel impelled to explore.

Keywords: physician-assisted suicide, euthanasia, hospice, palliative care, end-of-life

1. Introduction

"Can't the doctor just give me a pill to end it all now?" Some patients diagnosed with a terminal illness will feel unwilling to await natural death from their disease, especially if they anticipate that such waiting will lead to suffering, loss of control, loss of dignity, or a burden on loved ones. This chapter explores the options open to those who want to end life on their own schedule in 2022. Is there a pill? Does the doctor have it? How would that work? Is geography a factor? What choices are available to the reader today? This chapter addresses the choices available to cancer patients seeking "release" in 2022. Though the ethical issues involved in suicide and euthanasia generate rich, complex debate [1], this chapter reluctantly leaves that for another discussion, focusing instead on choices that a cancer patient can explore in 2022. Options involving a doctor are severely limited by geography and by the limitations inherent in medical practice, as we will discuss. Some readers may find that they have come here to choose a method of ending their lives, only to discover that choices are not limited to selecting a method of dying. Though we intend complete presentation of every method of dying reasonably available, the authors confess that we will be pleased every time readers make choices other than dying by their own hands.

2. Definitions

Clear definition facilitates discussion. All humans die. Most will experience *natural death*, death that occurs because of old age, disease, accident, or catastrophe. Though natural death is one of the choices for a cancer patient, this chapter focuses on those deaths hastened by human intervention. We set aside euphemisms increasingly used to obscure human intervention (Medical Assistance in Dying, Death with Dignity, and so forth) in favor of straightforward language and clear meaning. We define as *suicide* any death caused by injuring oneself with the intent to die. *Homicide* is the term used when one human takes the life of another. We examine *assisted suicide*, suicide undertaken with the aid of another person, and focus here primarily on the special circumstance termed *physician-assisted suicide (PAS)*, in which a physician assists a person seeking death, usually by writing a prescription for a lethal dose of drugs that the patient takes without assistance.

Euthanasia (literally, good dying) is the circumstance in which an action by one person produces the intentional death of another. In contrast with suicide, in which the person who takes the action is the one who dies, with euthanasia the person who takes the action (usually a doctor) performs this action on another person, who dies. *Passive euthanasia*, which is not our primary concern in this chapter, refers to removal of life-supporting medication or technical support, not often an issue for cancer patients. *Active euthanasia* involves one person taking an action that causes another to die (often by injection of a lethal preparation by a doctor). *Euthanasia* is *voluntary* when the person dying has requested it. Euthanasia on request is legal in some countries under limited conditions and is the only euthanasia to be considered in this chapter. *Involuntary euthanasia*, in which the person who dies has neither requested nor given consent to being killed, is never legal. In most of the world, involuntary euthanasia is considered homicide, or murder. Euthanasia without consent does occur, despite being illegal, and this is a source of intense concern and debate in countries that permit euthanasia.

In summary, *suicide* means I do something, and I die. *Physician assisted suicide* means I ask a doctor to prescribe lethal medication, and I take it by myself and die. *Voluntary euthanasia* means I ask a doctor to administer lethal medication, by drink or by injection, after which I die.

3. Why seek an end of life?

Many presume that patients with terminal illness endure great suffering without access to relief. This sad, desperate, and incomplete picture is commonly presented in lobbying campaigns that seek to legalize physician-assisted suicide. Actual reports from existing programs create a different picture. Oregon's 2020 report [2] on its PAS program, which presents the statistics for 2020, shows that 27% of patients were either in pain or worried that they would be in the future. Far more common reasons for seeking assisted suicide were loss of autonomy (93%), decreasing ability to participate in the activities that make life enjoyable (92%), and loss of dignity (68%). Ironically, even patients concerned about autonomy are required to sacrifice some of it to participate in a state's assisted suicide program. Participation usually requires pleading one's case to two separate doctors who will make the final judgment about whether to write a lethal prescription. The doctor—not the patient—decides whether a request for PAS will be honored. Use of the prescription itself remains autonomous; however, as no USA state exerts significant control over the prescribed lethal dose once it has been dispensed. Many patients inquire about assisted suicide but make other choices; many do not use the lethal prescription even when they have it in hand. In 2021, 383 people in Oregon received prescriptions for lethal medication, but only 219 are known to have died from ingesting the medication. One patient awoke after taking medication, 58 died without taking medication, and information on 106 patients is unclear, with 69 lost to follow-up [3].

4. Asking the doctor: it seems like a natural response

Facing the question of whether and how to seek an early end of life, some will fall back on their own resources, and others will seek help from the doctor. Why seek help from a doctor? Though ending one's life requires no collaboration with anyone at all, much less with a physician, the reality for most cancer patients is that they have been deeply involved in the medical care system for some time, from initial symptoms and diagnosis through rounds of chemotherapy, surgery, and radiation, or through rejection of those therapies as no longer valuable. Most cancer patients, therefore, have a close relationship with a physician, perhaps several, and are familiar with the medical care system. Thus, it follows that an initial search for relief might begin in that very system.

4.1 The limits of the doctor's power

Can a doctor simply prescribe a pill to end it all? No, not actually. A doctor is a surprisingly limited source of help in ending life early. Not only is there not a single pill that will instantly and painlessly end life, but also a doctor who assists with an intended suicide faces potential charges of homicide unless laws protect that participation. Though ending one's own life is not illegal, it is illegal to assist another person's suicide. The law views assistance in dying as helping kill the person. Only in the relatively few states or countries that have passed laws protecting doctors, pharmacists, and other professionals will doctors be able to help end life on request. At the present, doctors can help in 11 of the 50 states or districts in the USA, states with about one-sixth of the country's population. Nowhere in the USA can physicians perform euthanasia, legally administering lethal medication to end life. However, in those states with laws permitting PAS doctors can prescribe lethal medication for patients who can take it themselves. Elsewhere in the world, the Netherlands and Belgium have considerable experience in permitting physicians to produce death for patients by euthanasia or assisted suicide. Twelve countries around the world have passed laws protecting doctors who participate in assisted suicide or euthanasia; those countries are discussed extensively at the end of this chapter.

4.2 Doctors dealing death: a new phenomenon

Turning to a doctor as an agent of death is a relatively new phenomenon. In fact, doctors from the time of Hippocrates have given allegiance to an oath [4] in which they promise not to give poison to anybody when asked to do so, nor to suggest such a course. Doctors have portrayed themselves as healers, not dealers in death, and two thousand years of Hippocratic humility have consistently rejected the immense power inherent in allowing one human to cause the death of another [5]. Until relatively recently, physicians and society have agreed on the importance of keeping the power of death separate from the powers and privileges granted to physicians. In the past century, however, society has been willing in various locations to experiment with granting physicians the power to cause death. We are still early in a societal experiment, still recording the effects of unleashing that power.

4.3 The search for understanding

Killing any person, whether oneself or another person, has profound ethical implications, even when such an act is legal. This survey chapter is too short for complete ethical discussion. We have chosen to look at the situation in existence rather than questioning whether it should exist, reserving that discussion for another time. We acknowledge ending one's life is entirely possible in these times, with or without physician assistance. We have simply compiled in one place the information needed to begin a search for one's own answers to the question of what to do. How might one choose to end one's own life, and what consequences might follow? What choices deserve mention? We hope that some who have entered these discussions to choose a method for ending their lives will find that there are other choices, not obvious when the search began.

For readers making a serious attempt to understand options as fully as possible, and to choose whether to use any of those options, we strongly recommend additional reading and contemplation. Patients who want to end their own lives have access to a variety of means other than prescribed lethal overdoses of medication from physicians. Some of the means are messy, distressing, and uncertain (firearms, hanging, jumping from high places, poisoning) and some are little known and poorly publicized (inert gas inhalation, voluntary stopping of eating and drinking—VSED).

For serious seekers after truth, we recommend two books and a website. We do not agree with all the points of view in these sites, but we do believe that by and large the information is accurate. We believe that all three of these resources try to present detailed "how-to" discussions of techniques for ending life, coupled with careful and insightful discussions of not-so-appealing consequences of choosing any method, and thoughtful discussion of alternative choices.

4.4 Resources

4.4.1 Final Exit

Derek Humphrys' Final Exit is the classical "how-to" book, with detailed instructions on such non-doctor approaches as inert gas inhalation, and a careful rundown of preparations that must be made so paperwork and finances are in order. The book is full of caveats, legally sensitive, and a good book to have read at least twice for those who are increasingly serious. Many will find their curiosity satisfied and go no further [6].

4.4.2 The Peaceful Pill

Nitschke and Stewart's The Peaceful Pill is a meticulously detailed online book that's kept up to date (also available as hard copy that can become out of date).

Written by an Australian physician who has been a pioneer in this field, it discusses medications and methods in excruciating detail. It provides copious detail on how to find Nembutal (pentobarbital)—still considered the holy grail of the "peaceful pill" search (reliable, peaceful, and available). Finding the holy grail in 2022 requires veterinary connections, foreign sources, and a willingness to abandon being completely legal. Authors rate each method of suicide they discuss on Reliability, Peacefulness, and Availability. This book does not assume that a doctor will be involved in every death. The book provides considerable detail on suicide tourism in Switzerland [7].

4.4.3 Lostallhope.com

Lostallhope.com is a website constructed and maintained by a man who survived his own suicide attempt(s) years ago. It has an excellent and detailed review of approaches to suicide, as well as ranking by lethality, time to die, and agony. The author unblinkingly contrasts methods of suicide by country (USA 50% firearms, 25% hanging, 16% poisoning; versus United Kingdom [UK] 51% hanging, 20% drug poisoning), includes his own story and the stories of other survivors, discusses helpful reading, has a "help me" section, and lists several pages of people to call in crisis.

5. Permitting assisted suicide and euthanasia: laws that protect the doctor

Many people do not realize that suicide is legal almost everywhere in the world. Patients face no legal obstacles and need no legal protection to end their own lives or ask for assistance in doing so. A physician asked to assist, however, does need legal protection, as assisting may lead to a homicide charge. Legislation that "permits" PAS or euthanasia provides that legal protection, allowing a physician to provide lethal medication or even to administer it without being prosecuted for homicide. These laws generally protect physicians and other professionals, not patients. True, most laws have specific criteria for eligibility and a number of procedural steps, but those criteria seem primarily intended to demonstrate that physicians have conducted their due diligence and deserve protection.

6. Help from the doctor: hospice and palliative care

6.1 Hospice is open to all

Any patient diagnosed with terminal cancer and worried about the possibility of a declining quality of life deserves hospice care. Hospice in the USA is a Medicare benefit open to any Medicare subscriber within 6 months of the end of life. US hospice documents [8] say, "Hospice care is to relieve pain and other symptoms related to my terminal illness and related conditions ... The focus of hospice care is to provide comfort and support to both me and my family/caregivers." Mission Hospice, a typical US hospice, says that the primary goals of hospice care are to: "Relieve the physical, mental, emotional and spiritual suffering of our patients and those who care for them, promote the dignity and independence of our patients to the greatest extent possible, and support our patients and their families in finding personal fulfillment as they deal with end-of-life challenges." Palliative care—a generic term for medical care aimed at comfort and not cure—includes hospice care, but the generic term is not specifically limited to the terminally ill.

Hospice care is provided by specially trained nurses in homes or in facilities, with assistance from certified nursing assistants, social workers, spiritual counselors, and supervising hospice physicians. Most care is provided in the home. Hospice includes access to the best and most effective pain medication and symptom relief available anywhere, and hospice patients can be confident that pain or distress will be promptly treated and kept under control.

For several decades, hospice served primarily people with cancer, though that has shifted [9] in the last decade to the point where non-cancer diagnoses outnumber cancer four to one. In 2019 slightly more than half of Medicare patients who died were enrolled in hospice at the time of death. Average length of stay was 92.6 days, with median length of stay 18 days. Most of these days were in Routine Home Care, provided in a patient's own home or an assisted living facility, nursing home, or other congregate living facility. By 2019 there were 4840 Medicare certified hospices in operation.

The American Academy of Hospice and Palliative Medicine, which does not support legalizing PAS, recommends a 5-step approach to understanding requests for PAS, ending with a commitment to the patient to work toward a mutually acceptable solution for the patient's suffering. In situations where unacceptable suffering persists, they recommend discontinuation of potentially life-prolonging treatments (steroids, insulin, oxygen, dialysis, or artificial feeding or fluids). Consider voluntary stopping of oral intake (see VSED later in chapter). Finally, consider deep sedation (sometimes called, confusingly, palliative sedation), potentially to unconsciousness, if suffering remains intractable and severe [10].

6.2 How to choose a hospice

Most people have a choice of more than one hospice. How do they know which to choose? We suggest they interview representatives before making their choices, asking especially about how the hospice approaches pain relief, loss of function, anxiety, nausea, or other things they think might be troubling. Ask what some other patients have done to keep living lives that are rewarding. Ask especially about who will come to see a patient at night or on a weekend when the patient is having trouble or in pain. Will a nurse come see the patient? Is there a doctor on call, readily available? Is there a pharmacy readily available? Does the pharmacy deliver, so the patient will not be left alone while a caregiver is picking up medications?

6.3 The hospice inpatient unit

Ask whether the hospice has an inpatient unit or a place patients can go if they are too sick to be taken care of at home. Inpatient units in the United States are generally not for permanent residence, but for access to care when control of pain or symptoms needs full-time attention. Can a patient in overwhelming pain and distress receive deep sedation, in which patients are given as much medication as it takes to make them comfortable, all the while being carefully watched? True deep sedation, also called palliative sedation, for a suffering patient may require that the patient become unconscious before suffering is relieved. If the patient's pain and symptoms continue to need deep sedation to unconsciousness, comfort at this level may have the unintended effect of reducing a patient's ability to eat or drink. A deeply sedated patient may die painlessly of dehydration after several days of unconsciousness. Comfort, not death, is the aim of deep sedation, but death may come to a very ill patient who is comfortably sedated. Deep sedation, though rare, is best managed in an inpatient hospice unit, though unique circumstances might make it possible at home.

7. Help from the doctor: physician assisted suicide

7.1 The approval process

The goal of the process is for a patient to persuade a doctor to write a prescription for a lethal dose of medication that the patient can take without assistance. Those states and countries that have passed laws to protect physicians who help patients die have set out eligibility requirements that are quite similar. In general patients must be 18 or over, terminally ill with 6 months or less to live, able to give their own consent, able to administer medication to themselves, and able to request lethal medication on more than one occasion, usually with an additional request in writing. Switzerland does not require that the patient be terminally ill and does accept non-residents.

After the physician makes a prescription (sometimes after a mandated delay) the medication remains in the patient's keeping until used. Most laws suggest actions for the patient (tell the family, do not use the lethal dose in a public place, and return medication for safe disposal if unused) but none of these suggestions are attached to penalties for violation. In the USA a medical person is not required to attend death, and reports are requested but not mandated.

7.2 The medications

There is no single painless completely lethal pill that doctors can prescribe. No pharmacy has such a pill—governments would immediately prohibit distribution of any pill with such a high degree of lethality. A decade ago, doctors would have prescribed barbiturates, pentobarbital or secobarbital. However, in recent years manufacturers have removed some medications from the market (no pharmaceutical manufacturer wants to be known as the provider of death medications). When barbiturates were available, a pharmacist would provide enough medication to make a lethal dose if taken all at once. That might require, say, 3 months of one-a-day capsules that would have to be opened, dumped into a slurry with something like applesauce to disguise the bitter taste, and eaten all at once to avoid falling asleep before a lethal dose is ingested, perhaps to awaken the next day still alive—with a headache. All this is simply to say that these methods are neither easy nor foolproof; many things can go wrong. Self-medication to death can be a risky, sometimes unsuccessful business.

More often now, doctors prescribe a mixture of three to five medications intended to work together to provide death. Oregon's 2021 data summary [11] shows that although barbiturates were the most common medications through about 2018, various combinations of diazepam, digoxin, morphine sulfate, and amitriptyline, with or without phenobarbital, have been introduced and evolved, with replacement of one drug by another and variations in dose of each ingredient. The law does not specify the medication, but simply permits a lethal prescription. Since there is no laboratory in which a physician can test a new lethal mixture on humans, there is a real possibility that a new mixture will not work as well as hoped when given to a real patient.

Although doctors who assist are committed to providing painless and effective death, an untested mixture might lead to an unsuccessful suicide attempt, or it might lead to an attempt marred by suffering and agony, perhaps without a doctor even present.

Assisted suicide, by definition, means that nobody but the patient is supposed to administer medications. Physically assisting by, for example, forcing more medication into a semiconscious patient, could lead to being charged with a felony. It is not possible without risking prosecution to give more medication if the patient is already unconscious and cannot take more medication unassisted. In the rare countries that permit physicians to provide euthanasia by administering lethal medications, assisted suicide becomes much less common than euthanasia. When doctors give lethal medication, they do not stop until the patient is dead. Moreover, they can give intravenous medications that work almost instantaneously, as in the operating room, rather than prescribing massive doses of oral medications that may work slowly, may produce incomplete effects if doses are too low, may be inappropriate medications in the first place, or may cause vomiting and loss of medication that cannot be replaced because the patient is already falling asleep.

7.3 Ethical issues

Ethical issues that arise with assisted suicide concern selection of appropriate candidates, protection of candidates susceptible to coercion, custody of lethal medication once dispensed, accommodation for patients incapable of self-administration, and accuracy of tracking results. Patients with mental illness are presumed to be screened out, but only two states require mental health screening. Other states only suggest it. As mentioned, not every lethal dose is consumed, and no current mechanism tracks all the medication dispensed. There is no requirement for medical attendance at death, and no firm requirement for reporting events during medication administration. As written, the laws do not accommodate patients with physical disabilities that make self-administration impossible (quadriplegia, neurodegenerative diseases).

8. Help from the doctor: euthanasia

8.1 The approval process

Countries that permit euthanasia are rare, but their criteria for eligibility for euthanasia share some elements. Patients who qualify to have doctors end their lives are generally required to be adults, capable of sound decisions, free of coercion, and suffering some sort of grievous and irreversible medical condition. In Canada, death needs to be foreseeable. Belgium requires constant and unbearable suffering that cannot be alleviated. Luxembourg requires a grave and incurable condition. Spain requires a serious or incurable illness or a chronic or incapacitating condition that causes intolerable suffering. Colombia requires a terminal illness but has expanded its reach to nonterminal illness such as chronic obstructive pulmonary disease or amyotrophic lateral sclerosis.

The Netherlands has experienced legalized euthanasia for longer than any other country and has broadened their criteria over the years. The Netherlands permits euthanasia for terminally ill children as young as 12 years old. In addition, in the Groningen Protocol [12], the Netherlands has authorized newborn euthanasia for children born with unbearable suffering, if parents, their physician, and an independent physician agree. Dutch law requires hopeless and unbearable suffering, but a provision that would allow assisted death without a terminal illness for a person who feels they have completed life has been much discussed.

8.2 The medications

Medication given by a physician to end life can be given as a drink or can be administered intravenously. The drink is usually a strong barbiturate potion (10 grams or more), often preceded by an anti-nausea drug. Intravenous medications mirror those used to start a surgical anesthetic—a barbiturate when thiopental was easily available, and now more frequently propofol, followed by a paralyzing drug after the patient has lost consciousness. Though the medications may seem identical, the euthanasia protocol would be to give the medications and allow the patient to become unconscious, stop breathing, and die of oxygen shortage. The euthanasia patient never awakens. An operating room protocol, on the other hand, might use the same medications but would supplement the breathing and provide oxygen to keep the brain alive, monitoring every breath and every heartbeat to keep the patient stable, administering more anesthetic agent in the IV or by inhalation as needed for the patient to remain unconscious until time to awaken.

8.3 Ethical questions

Beyond those questions inherent in giving a doctor the freedom to take an action that ends a patient's life, questions around euthanasia tend to be of the "slippery slope" variety. That is, if it is permissible to end life for a 12-year-old, how about an unusually mature 10- or 11-year-old? What about a patient who asks for euthanasia when of sound mind, but now has such significant dementia that the patient can no longer confirm consent? If voluntary euthanasia is permitted, how about those cases where the patient can no longer consent but those charged with the patient's welfare are sure that the patient would have wanted life to end?

9. What can be done to shorten life? Using one's own resources

9.1 Ending life without a doctor

9.1.1 Why we die

Man is an obligate aerobe [13]. Every cell in our bodies depends on oxygen for the metabolic processes that sustain life. Although some cells such as skeletal muscles can function anaerobically (without oxygen) for a short time, accumulating an oxygen debt by forming lactic acid to be broken down when oxygen is available again, the brain cannot. The brain requires a continuing and largely uninterrupted supply of oxygen, and therefore of the blood that carries oxygen. All methods of producing death that we discuss as methods of suicide or euthanasia interrupt oxygen to the brain. Lethal doses of sedatives may stop breathing, may allow the airway to obstruct so air exchange ceases, and may themselves stop the heart. Major trauma (e.g., gunshot, car crash, and fall from a height) may destroy the brain or heart, or more likely will lead to blood loss that eventually leaves the heart running on empty, with no oxygenated blood to send to the brain. Hanging or strangulation stops blood flow to the brain. Poisons may stop the heart. Inhaling an inert gas displaces oxygen from the lungs, leading to oxygen lack, rapid unconsciousness, and rapid death of brain and then heart.

9.2 Suicide in the USA: grading the methods

Suicide without physician assistance accounts for about 1.5% of deaths worldwide [14]. Rates vary by country, from as high as 53 deaths per 100,000 population in Greenland to as few as 3 per 100,000 in Peru [15]. In the USA, rates vary by state from a high of 29.6 per 100,000 in Montana to a low of 6.1 per 100,000 in the District of Columbia [16].

"lostallhope.com" has an extensive listing of methods of killing oneself, evaluated according to lethality (99% for shotgun to head, 6% for cutting wrists), time required (1.4 min for shotgun to chest, 456 min for overdose of nonprescription drugs), and agony (3.75 for explosives, 95 for setting fire to self). Those seriously evaluating methods for ending their own lives may want to examine this list of options, none of which require assistance from a physician.

Not included in this list is any accounting of the effect on bystanders, on those who find the person who has accomplished suicide, and on families. In general, some of the most effective and available methods are those frequently used, with lifelong effects on survivors and those left to clean up after a violent death.

9.3 Less easily available methods

Several methods of ending life are less violent.

9.3.1 Medications

Medications are extensively dealt with in the three references above. In general, non-prescription overdoses have a high risk of failure. However, prescription overdoses not officially provided by assisted suicide programs also fail at a high rate. Opioids (narcotics) are often used by those who want to bypass physician consultation and use materials available at home. Some cancer patients will have massive doses of opioids at home, and some will be encouraged to take huge doses of these medications as a method of inducing respiratory arrest and death. Be warned! Patients who have been taking opioids for pain relief will be refractory to the respiratory effects of even massive doses of drugs and will very likely commit themselves to several days of deep sleep and a distressing wake-up in the midst of continuing life. Worse, many will have communicated their plans to family, who may panic on discovering that the intended lethal dose is not working, taking actions to bring death to their loved one that will lead to their having committed homicide, whether charged with it or not.

Poisons, such as insecticides, are also extensively dealt with in the references. All such methods have a high risk of failure and continued life with injury and cannot be recommended for consideration.

9.3.2 Inert gas inhalation

Inhaling inert gas (helium, argon, or nitrogen) is a painless, effective, and very accessible means of dying. Both books cited above describe technique and equipment in detail. Although doctors could recommend this setup as more effective than the medications they prescribe, they do not. Doctors prescribe medication, for the most part, and do not think of inhalation. Anesthesiologists think of inhalation but are generally not involved in assisting suicides.

"Painless" dying occurs when the brain stops functioning first, and then the heart. This can happen with drugs that abolish consciousness first, then stop breathing, then stop the heart. Eliminating oxygen from the air being breathed can also abolish consciousness first and then lead to rapid death of brain and heart, all with no poison or toxin at all. How can that happen?

In normal breathing we inhale air containing 21% oxygen, 78% nitrogen, 1% other gases, and very little carbon dioxide (0.04%). Since the body uses oxygen and produces carbon dioxide in its metabolic processes, the exhaled air after exchange in the lungs contains less oxygen (17%) and much more carbon dioxide (4%, about 100 times as much). Nitrogen is still there unchanged, but exhaled water vapor has diluted it a bit.

Breathing is automatic, generally. Our respiratory control center notices that carbon dioxide is rising and triggers a breath. Our body's breathing control mechanism is very sensitive to little rises in carbon dioxide. Too much carbon dioxide sends a loud alarm signal to the brain to defend the airway at any expense, because if carbon dioxide is rising something has gone frightfully wrong with breathing. Anybody who has breathed for even a short time into a paper bag, rebreathing carbon dioxide as it builds up, knows the desperate feeling of suffocation that shortly makes us take the bag away and breathe fresh air again.

Unlike too much carbon dioxide, the body has very weak alarms for too little oxygen. Rather, low oxygen produces primarily sleepiness and then unconsciousness. A pilot whose oxygen supply has been interrupted, or a shipyard worker who has unknowingly entered a chamber flushed with nitrogen that has displaced all the oxygen, feels no distress but keeps on breathing normally until unconsciousness sets in. Breathing is perfectly normal, even when there is no oxygen in the air, so the carbon dioxide level stays normal and the carbon dioxide alarm is never set off. A single lungful of an inert gas, such as helium, can produce rapid hypoxia (oxygen shortage) and rapid unconsciousness with no sensation of being short of breath. Anybody who has inhaled the entire content of a helium balloon and held their breath can attest to the rapid onset of light-headedness and impending loss of consciousness. Usually, the person breathing from the balloon would lose consciousness, drop the balloon, and be restored by breathing oxygen-containing room air, since breathing would not stop. If, however, an entire balloon of helium surrounded the person's head so that breathing pure helium would continue, death would rapidly follow, and the person who dies would only have been aware of falling peacefully asleep, breathing normally.

This phenomenon is the basis of a suicide technique known as "inert gas inhalation." An inert gas is one that has no toxic or anesthetic properties of its own but simply displaces oxygen in pure gas breathing. Nitrogen, argon, and helium are the commonest examples of inert gases. Breathing from a large plastic bag (think turkey bag) filled with one of these gases placed around the head and face, sealed loosely at the neck, will produce unconsciousness within one to three breaths, and death within minutes. All inert gases can be purchased or rented from gas suppliers, welding shops, or even toy stores that carry balloon supplies (though helium that has been blended with 20% oxygen would not work for this purpose). Inert gas inhalation requires some preparation and some purchase of supplies but does not require the presence of another (though recommended). Most importantly, it does not require a prescription or the participation of a doctor. It leaves no telltale signs, creates no distressing mess, and (especially in the case of nitrogen) is generally undetectable on autopsy. These features make it the technique of choice for those looking for a painless, low-stress approach to suicide that does not require requesting a physician's participation.

9.3.3 Voluntarily stopping eating and drinking (VSED)

Since eating and drinking are essential to life, one way to control life is to control eating and drinking. Stopping eating and drinking, it can be argued, is ethically permissible in the same way that foregoing life-sustaining treatment is permissible. In fact, failing to honor a competent patient's refusal of food and drink could lead to an attempt at force feedings, with a nasogastric tube and restraints, a complete violation of a patient's dignity and autonomy. The Supreme Court of the United States of America has affirmed the right of a capable individual to refuse any unwanted treatment [17], even if that refusal results in death. Dr. Timothy Quill has written an up-to-date and complete book with answers to virtually all questions about VSED [18].

Death usually occurs within 1–3 weeks of starting a fast, depending on the patient's physical condition. Dehydrated, cachectic patients decline in a shorter time than obese, well-hydrated patients. This is not a process for a solo individual—as the fasting person declines, round-the-clock attention becomes necessary. Further, general agreement of family and caregivers gives peace and support for a process that is not easy every minute.

The first few days of fasting may find the patient awake and responsive, able to reminisce and to examine in detail the course chosen. As dehydration progresses, the patient becomes sleepier and more lethargic, eventually becoming completely unresponsive before death. Though pain and discomfort are not common, good palliative support is invaluable.

Once committed, most patients want the process to move as quickly as possible. The number one bit of advice is to take no fluids at all, including fluids taken with medication. Even a little bit of water every day may prolong the dying process by days. Most patients will complete their fasting journey in several days to a week [19]. Those who take longer are almost always taking some sort of fluids. In a Dutch study of the VSED experience of patients of 708 family physicians median time to death was 7 days; 8% had a prolonged process of 14 days or more [20].

VSED is particularly well suited to patients with gastrointestinal obstruction or difficulty swallowing, or those with sufficient control to deal with discomfort in early stages. For some, VSED has the appeal of being an entirely natural process that needs no medication or instrumentation. It is also legal and effective even in states where assisted suicide is not protected. Although patient experience is better if those in the environment are supportive, the process depends entirely on an individual decision. VSED is supported by most hospices and is an extension of the end-of-life process that many experience, with stopping eating and drinking as death approaches.

10. Get your financial house in order

Do not forget about getting your financial house in order—will, living will, POA selection, accounts in order, insurances discovered, etc. Having all the details of your accounts, beneficiaries, funeral wishes and such in one place will make things easier for your heirs and those who are tasked with planning and executing your wishes. Use a simple book where you can fill in the essential information, or you can provide your attorney's information if your trust and/or will is there.

DOI: http://dx.doi.org/10.5772/intechopen.105989

11. Geographic limitations on physician assistance

See **Table 1**.

11.1 Countries in which euthanasia and physician-assisted suicide are legal

11.1.1 Netherlands

Euthanasia and physician-assisted suicide were legalized in the Netherlands in 2002 for Dutch citizens over 12 years old, in an act that made physicians exempt from criminal responsibility if they practiced under a set of conditions established by the law. Newborns have been eligible to be euthanized since 2004 under the Groningen Protocol if they are believed to have unbearable suffering and parents, the child's physician, and an independent physician agree to the procedure. In 2020 the Dutch announced plans to extend euthanasia to terminally ill children between the ages of one and 12. Euthanasia tourism is not possible: citizenship is not the issue. The treating physician who will vouch for the patient must be in the Netherlands. A patient cannot be treated outside the Netherlands and receive euthanasia in the Netherlands. Euthanasia rates have risen from just under 2% of all deaths in 2002 to just over 4% in 2019 [22].

11.1.2 Belgium

Belgium legalized PAS and euthanasia in 2002 for "competent" adults and emancipated minors suffering from "constant and unbearable physical or mental suffering that cannot be alleviated." Patients do NOT need to be suffering from terminal illness. The law was extended to minors in 2014. The Analysis of the 2020 Commission Report [23] asserted that 954 reported assisted deaths in 2010 had increased to 2656 by 2019, an increase of 267% in 9 years. The main conditions generating requests were cancer or polypathology unlikely to improve; no unemancipated minor euthanasia was recorded.

11.1.3 Luxembourg

Luxembourg became the third country in Europe to legalize euthanasia and physician-assisted suicide with a law that went into effect in 2009. Doctors have legal immunity from prosecution and lawsuits if they perform euthanasia or PAS for a patient with a grave and incurable condition who has asked repeatedly for the procedure. Luxembourg also requires palliative care and paid leave for relatives of terminally ill family members. In all cases, before euthanasia or assisted suicide can be performed, the doctor must fulfill certain formal and procedural conditions (e.g., conduct several interviews with the patient, etc.) [24].

Patients who live elsewhere but have a physician in Luxembourg may record end-of-life wishes and plans in their medical file. Luxembourg attaches no stipulations of residency or nationality to placing this information in one's medical file. However, the physician must have been caring for the patient for a long, uninterrupted period. Minors, persons of legal age under guardianship or protection, and legally incapable persons may not legally request euthanasia or assisted suicide, nor may their parents, guardians or trustees make such a request on their behalf.

Country	Assisted suicide?	Euthanasia
Belgium	Legal	Legal
Canada	Legal	Legal
Luxembourg	Legal	Legal
Netherlands	Legal	Legal
Spain	Legal	Legal
Australia	Legal in all states but Northern Territory and Australian Capital Territory	Legal in all states but Northern Territory and Australian Capital Territory)
Colombia	Illegal	Legal
Austria	Legal	Illegal
Finland	Legal	Illegal
Germany	Legal	Illegal
New Zealand	Legal	Illegal
Switzerland	Legal	Illegal
Japan	Unclear	Unclear
South Africa	Unclear	Unclear
United States	Illegal (legal in OR, WA, CA, HI, NM, MT, ME, VT, CO, NJ, DC)	Illegal
China	Illegal	Illegal
Denmark	Illegal	Illegal
France	Illegal	Illegal
India	Illegal	Illegal
Ireland	Illegal	Illegal
Israel	Illegal	Illegal
Italy	Illegal	Illegal
Mexico	Illegal	Illegal
Norway	Illegal	Illegal
Philippines	Illegal	Illegal
Russia	Illegal	Illegal
Sweden	Illegal	Illegal
Turkey	Illegal	Illegal
United Kingdom	Illegal	Illegal
Uruguay	Illegal	Illegal

Table 1.
Countries allowing assisted suicide or euthanasia, 2022 [21].

The sixth biennial report by the National Commission for Control and Evaluation [25], published in March 2021, records 16 cases of euthanasia in 2019 (twice the 8 cases in 2018) and 25 cases in 2020. Total cases from 2009 to 2020 were 112. Lethal injection was the mode for all but occasional rare cases of oral ingestion of a barbiturate. In 2020 the Commission approved the first euthanasia of a 96-year-old man claiming "fatigue of life," citing the Belgian practice.

11.1.4 Canada

Canada decriminalized suicide in 1972 but retained a provision prohibiting assisted suicide until it was struck down in 2015 by the Supreme Court of Canada, which gave the Canadian Parliament 1 year to pass a law legalizing and regulating physician-assisted suicide and perhaps euthanasia. Bill C-14 [26] passed the Senate in 2016, making assisted suicide and possibly euthanasia legal. The Court was unclear about the distinction between PAS and euthanasia, but Bill C-14 states that "medical assistance in dying (MAID) means (a) the administering by a medical practitioner or nurse practitioner of a substance to a person, at their request, that causes death; or (b) the prescribing or providing by a medical practitioner or nurse practitioner of a substance to a person, at their request, so that they may self-administer the substance and in doing so, cause their own death." These provisions apply to citizens or permanent residents of Canada, at least 18 years old, who have a "grievous and irremediable medical condition." To be eligible for MAID [27] in Canada, a person must be at least 18 years of age and be eligible for publicly funded health care services in Canada. By November 2020, more than 13,000 Individuals [28] nearing the end of life had been voluntarily euthanized as a result of this bill. In 2020, 2.5% of deaths in Canada were due to MAID. In March 2023, Canada is set to become one of the few nations allowing medical aid in dying (MAID) for people with afflictions that are solely mental, such as depression, schizophrenia, bipolar disorder, personality disorder, PTSD, or other mental affliction. In March 2021, Bill C-7 [29] made changes to the eligibility criteria, removing the "reasonably foreseeable death" criterion. As of March 17, 2023, MAID will be available to capable adults whose sole underlying condition is a mental illness.

Canada's MAID law says that intolerable suffering is wholly subjective and personal. Unlike the Netherlands, a doctor does not have to agree. Suffering is what the person says it is. Under those criteria, the Council of Canadian Academies suggests that Canada could become the most permissive jurisdiction in the world with respect to MAID and mental illness [30].

11.1.5 Spain

The fifth country to legalize both PAS and euthanasia, Spain wrote a "death with dignity" bill in 2011 that allowed passive euthanasia, the removal of treatment or life-sustaining machinery. Ten years later, Spain's parliament legalized both active euthanasia and PAS for Spanish citizens and legal residents who suffer from a "serious or incurable illness" or a "chronic or incapacitating condition" that causes "intolerable suffering" [31]. The person seeking death must make two requests, 15 days apart, in writing, and must be found "fully aware and conscious."

11.2 A country in which euthanasia alone is legal

11.2.1 Colombia

Though Colombia's Constitutional Court appeared to legalize euthanasia in 1997 when it ruled that physicians could not be prosecuted for assisting with suicide, legalization awaited Health Ministry released guidelines that were not released until 2015. In 2021 the Court recognized that the procedure should be available to persons with degenerative illnesses as well as terminal illnesses. On March 9, 2018, Colombia passed a resolution permitting euthanasia for children [32]. Children under 14 require parental consent, but those over 14 may give their own consent even if parents disagree.

11.3 Countries in which physician-assisted suicide alone is legal

11.3.1 Austria

In 2020 Austria's constitutional court ruled that banning assisted suicide violated fundamental rights. Effective in January 2022, two doctors review each case (one must be a palliative care physician), and a 12-week waiting period applies unless the patient is terminal. Austria reported 1160 suicides in 2019, 68 fewer than in 2018. Of those, 907 were men, 253 were women, making suicide the leading causes of unnatural death in Austria.

11.3.2 Finland

Finland's National Advisory Board on Social Welfare and Health Care Ethics (ETENE) created a statement released in 2021 asserting that assisted suicide is not a crime in Finland [33]. This was to involve placing medication within reach of a patient but requiring the patient to take the deadly dose himself/herself. The group took no position on legalization of euthanasia but suggested that discussion should continue.

11.3.3 Germany

Germany legalized physician-assisted suicide in 2015 when performed on "an individual basis out of altruistic motives," but commercial euthanasia and suicide business were out. In 2020 a high court overturned the ban on professionally provided assisted suicide [34]. There is an ongoing debate in Germany about how to settle the issue, but regardless of that parliament cannot overturn the decision of the constitutional court. Assisted suicide will remain legal in Germany under certain, specific circumstances, but the decision for how it will be regulated now lies with the parliament.

11.3.4 New Zealand

After numerous unsuccessful legislative attempts, a nationwide vote in 2020 legalized physician-assisted suicide, effective November 7, 2021. New Zealand's Ministry of Health maintains an informative web site [35] that answers most potential questions about what it calls its Assisted Dying Service; noncitizens are not eligible to apply for the service. In the 5 months preceding March 31, 2022, 206 people applied for assisted dying. As of March 31, 66 people had already obtained an assisted death, 59 were still trying, and 81 people had not persisted (they were ineligible, they withdrew, or they died) [36].

11.3.5 Switzerland

Euthanasia is illegal. Article 114 of the Penal Code of Switzerland forbids causing the death of a person even in the face of genuine and repeated requests. Article 115 forbids assisting with suicide for "selfish motives." Assisted suicide is permissible if the person assisting has good intentions and does not actually administer the medication that leads to death. Dignitas clinic [37] in Forch performs "accompanied suicides." Dignitas provides detailed information in their brochure, which emphasizes that the process is detailed, time-consuming, and expensive. Novelist Amy Bloom has written about her husband's death in Switzerland [38] and has been interviewed on NPR about that experience [39].

11.4 Countries in which the status of PAS and euthanasia is unclear

11.4.1 Japan

Despite the absence of specific laws banning euthanasia, physician-assisted suicide is a criminal offense. A District Court in 1995 found a physician guilty of homicide for injecting lethal drugs at a patient's request and set out four conditions to be met for active euthanasia to be legal. The same court in 2005 found a physician guilty of homicide for removing an endotracheal tube and giving a muscle relaxant without the patient's permission, a conviction upheld in 2007 by a court critical of the lower court's rules but unwilling to produce new ones. The Supreme Court declined to hear the case.

11.4.2 South Africa

The South African Law Commission in 1997 produced a draft law that would have legalized both euthanasia and PAS, but the report was ignored, and a law never passed. In 2015 a terminally ill lawyer asked that his physician be allowed to assist with his suicide, but the court's supportive ruling was not read until the lawyer had already died, leaving the scope of the ruling unclear.

11.5 Countries in which individual states permit PAS or euthanasia despite country-wide bans

11.5.1 Australia

Despite previous countrywide bans on both euthanasia and PAS, the state of Victoria passed a law in 2017 that allowed doctors to prescribe lethal drugs for self-administration by terminally ill patients; the law also allowed doctors to administer the medications if the patient is unable to do so themselves. Western Australia followed in 2019, followed in 2021 by Tasmania, Queensland, and South Australia. Parliament will be under pressure to permit legalization of assisted dying in the Northern Territory and in the Australian Capital Territory.

11.5.2 United States of America

The USA holds euthanasia illegal everywhere, in every state. However, 10 of 50 states and the District of Columbia have laws protecting physicians involved in physician-assisted suicide if procedures are followed. These states will be examined in detail in the subsequent section.

11.6 Countries in which physician-assisted suicide or euthanasia are illegal

Table 1 lists several specific countries in which PAS or euthanasia are not protected. The fact that a country is not on the list attests only to lack of information and does not imply that PAS or euthanasia might be legal in unlisted countries.

11.7 A more detailed look at USA states in which PAS is protected

USA states that permit physician assisted suicide have very similar laws, all based on the same core template espoused by advocates in Oregon. Montana is an exception, as its protection is based on a court ruling in 2009 which held that consent could be a defense against a charge of homicide in a case of PAS. No legislative or regulatory steps have been completed there (**Table 2**).

All states require that candidates be at least 18 and diagnosed with a terminal illness that limits life expectancy to 6 months or less. All states require two oral and one written request for services except for New Mexico. All states protect patients' insurance and contracts. Mental health consultation is required in Hawaii and Colorado and is left up to screening physicians elsewhere. All states require a second "consultant" physician who confirms the diagnosis and the patient's capability of giving their own consent.

Montana, on the other hand, having arrived at assisted suicide by a court decision, has no legislative framework to follow, and no reporting structure.

State	Date passed	Residency required?	Minimum age	Months until expected death	Number of requests to provider
California	2015	Yes	18	6 or fewer	2 oral, 15 d apart, one written
Colorado	2016	Yes	18	6 or fewer	2 oral, 15 d apart, one written
District of Columbia	2016	Yes	18	6 or fewer	2 oral, 15 d apart, one written
Hawaii	2018	Yes	18	6 or fewer	2 oral, 20 d apart, one written
Maine	2019	Yes	18	6 or fewer	2 oral, 20 d apart, one written
Montana	2009	Yes	No legal protocol	No legal protocol	No legal protocol
New Jersey	2019	Yes	18	6 or fewer	2 oral, 15 d apart, one written
New Mexico	2021	Yes	18	6 or fewer	One written request (state form)
Oregon	1994	No (starting 2022)	18	6 or fewer	Two oral, one written
Vermont	2013	Yes	18	6 or fewer	2 oral, 15 d apart, one written
Washington	2008	Yes	18	6 or fewer	2 oral, 15 d apart, one written

Table 2.
States of the USA in which physician-assisted suicide is protected.

A recent report, from 2019, says that 4249 prescriptions for lethal medication have been written since 1998 in US states, and that 66.3% of these patients have used the drugs to end their lives. Of note for this chapter, 63.1% of these patients had cancer [40].

11.7.1 California

ABX2-12 End of Life Option Act [41], was signed into Law Oct. 5, 2015, and became effective June 9, 2016.

Contact California Department of Health, **Phone:** 916-558-1784.

Patient eligibility: As with other states, candidates must be 18 or older, residents of the state, and able to make their own decisions and communicate them. A patient must have a terminal illness with a life expectancy of 6 months or less but must still be physically and mentally capable of self-administering the prescribed lethal medication without assistance. **Physician requirements:** The doctor must diagnose a terminal illness with a life expectancy of 6 months or less. This must be confirmed by a second consulting doctor, who is also expected to certify that the patient can make and communicate health care decisions. If either doctor questions the patient's ability to make judgments, the patient must be referred for a psychological examination. The attending doctor must inform the patient of alternatives, including hospice, palliative care, and pain management options. **Patient request timeline:** First oral request to doctor, 15-day waiting period, second oral request to doctor along with written request. **Other:** Patient's insurance is protected from being affected by patient's decision to "use law." Doctors and health care systems have choice about whether to participate. Non-English speakers are to have translators available. Pharmacists cannot be prosecuted for filling lethal prescriptions.

11.7.2 Colorado

Proposition 106: End of Life Options Act [42], came from voters Nov. 8, 2016 (65% in favor), became **Effective:** Jan. 2017.

Colorado Department of Public Health & Environment **Phone:** 303-692-2000; **Email:** cdphe.information@state.co.us

Patient eligibility: As with other states, candidates must be 18 or older, residents of the state, and able to make their own decisions and communicate them. They must have made requests voluntarily. A patient must have a terminal illness with a life expectancy of 6 months or less. **Physician requirements:** The doctor must diagnose a terminal illness with a life expectancy of 6 months or less, confirm the patient's capacity to make and communicate medical decisions, and confirm residency. Diagnosis must be confirmed by a second consulting doctor, who is also expected to confirm competency. The doctor must refer the patient to a licensed mental health professional. The doctor must discuss diagnosis, prognosis, feasible alternatives, and risks of taking lethal medication, as well as possibility of choosing not to use it. The doctor should tell the patient to notify next of kin, and request that medication not be taken in a public place. **Patient request timeline:** First oral request to doctor, 15-day waiting period, second oral request to doctor along with written request. **Other:** Patient's insurance is protected from being affected by patient's decision to "use law." Doctors and health care systems have choice about whether to participate.

11.7.3 District of Columbia

DC ACT 21-577 *Death with Dignity Act of 2016* [43], **Signed into Law** Dec. 19, 2016, **Effective Date:** Feb. 18, 2017.

DC Department of Health **Phone:** 202-442-5955 **Email:** doh@dc.gov

Patient eligibility: As with other states, candidates must be 18 or older, residents of the District, and able to make their own decisions and communicate them. A patient must have a terminal illness with a life expectancy of 6 months or less. **Physician requirements:** The doctor must diagnose a terminal illness with a life expectancy of 6 months or less. This must be confirmed by a second consulting doctor, who is also expected to certify that the patient can make and communicate health care decisions. If either doctor questions the patient's ability to make judgments, the patient must be referred for a psychological examination. The attending doctor must inform the patient of alternatives, including palliative care, hospice, and pain management options. **patient request Timeline:** First oral request to doctor, 15-day waiting period, second oral request to doctor along with written request before second request, then 48-hour waiting period before drugs dispensed. **Other:** Patient's insurance is protected from being affected by patient's decision to "use law."

11.7.4 Hawaii

HB 2739, Hawai'i Our Care, Our Choice Act [44] **signed into Law** Apr. 5, 2018, **effective Date** January 1, 2019.

Hawaii Department of Health **Phone:** 808-586-4400, **Email:** webmail@doh.hawaii.gov

Highlights of the law (use Hyperlink to see entire law):

Patient eligibility: As with other states, candidates must be 18 or older, residents of the state, and able to make their own decisions and communicate them. A patient must have a terminal illness with a life expectancy of 6 months or less. **Physician requirements:** The doctor must diagnose a terminal illness with a life expectancy of 6 months or less. This must be confirmed by a second consulting doctor, who is also expected to certify that the patient can make and communicate health care decisions. A counselor must confirm that the patient is capable and not suffering from depression or impaired decision-making ability. The attending doctor must inform the patient of alternatives, including palliative care, hospice, and pain management options. **Patient request timeline:** First oral request to doctor, 20-day waiting period, second oral request to doctor along with witnessed written request before second request; 48 h to prescription. **Other:** The patient can withdraw request at any time and is not required to fill the prescription. Patient's insurance is protected from being affected by patient's decision to "use law."

11.7.5 Maine

HP 948, An Act to Enact the Maine Death with Dignity Act [45] **signed into Law** June 12, 2019, **effective Date** September 19, 2019.

Note: Maine's law indicates that it does not legalize "assisted suicide," but states that the act must be referred to as "obtaining and administering life-ending medication" in state reports. Note that this does not alter the action for which the physician is protected.

Maine Department of Health and Human Services **Phone:** 207-287-3707.

Patient eligibility: As with other states, candidates must be 18 or older, residents of the state, and able to make their own decisions and communicate them. A patient must have a terminal illness with a life expectancy of 6 months or less but must still be physically and mentally capable of self-administering the prescribed lethal medication without assistance. **Physician requirements:** The doctor must diagnose a terminal illness with a life expectancy of 6 months or less and judge the patient mentally capable of making an informed, voluntary decision. This must be confirmed by a second consulting doctor, who is also expected to certify that the patient can make and communicate health care decisions and is acting voluntarily. If either doctor questions the patient's ability to make judgments, the patient must be referred for a psychological examination. The attending doctor must discuss diagnosis and prognosis, and inform the patient of alternatives, including palliative care, hospice, and pain management options, as well as risks of taking lethal medication and possibility of not taking it. Patient is to be requested to notify next of kin, and not take medication in a public place. **Patient request timeline:** First oral request to doctor, 15-day waiting period, second oral request to doctor along with written request signed at least 15 days after first request; 48 h to prescription. **Other:** The patient may withdraw the request at any time and is not required to fill the prescription. Patient's insurance is protected from being affected by patient's decision to "use law." No will, contract, or other agreement can interfere with patient's use of law.

11.7.6 Montana

Montana First Judicial District Court: *Baxter v. Montana* [46]

Court ruling date: Dec. 5, 2008, in favor of plaintiffs.

Plaintiffs (four physicians and a dying patient) asked court to establish constitutional right "to receive and provide aid in dying." Judge ruled that a terminally ill, competent patient has a legal right to die with dignity under Article II, Sections 4 and 10 of the Montana Constitution, including a right to "use the assistance of his physician to obtain a prescription for a lethal dose of medication that the patient may take on his own if and when he decides to terminate his life." Judge further held that this right "includes protection of that patient's physician from liability under the State's homicide statutes."

State Supreme Court: **Baxter v. Montana**

Decided: Dec. 31, 2009, in favor of plaintiffs 5-4.

The Attorney General of Montana appealed the ruling above to the Montana Supreme Court, which said, "we find no indication in Montana law that physician aid in dying provided to terminally ill, mentally competent adult patients is against public policy." Therefore, the physician who assists is shielded from criminal liability *by the patient's consent*.

No legal protocol is in place.

Despite multiple legislative attempts since 2009, neither laws nor regulations dealing with assisted suicide have been put in place in Montana.

11.7.7 New Jersey

Bill A1504 Aid in Dying for the Terminally Ill Act [47] signed into Law Apr. 12, 2019, e**ffective Date** Aug. 1, 2019.

State of New Jersey Department of Health **Phone:** 800-367-6543.

Patient eligibility: As with other states, candidates must be 18 or older, residents of the state, and able to make their own decisions and communicate them. A patient must have a terminal illness with a life expectancy of 6 months or less. **Physician requirements:** The doctor must diagnose a terminal illness with a life expectancy of 6 months or less. This must be confirmed by a second consulting doctor, who is also expected to certify that the patient can make and communicate health care decisions. If either doctor questions the patient's ability to make judgments, the patient must be referred for a psychological examination. The attending doctor must inform the patient of alternatives, including hospice, palliative care, and pain management options. The physician should request that the patient notify next of kin. **Patient request timeline:** First oral request to doctor, 15-day waiting period, second oral request to doctor along with written request; 48 h to dispensing. **Other:** Patient's ability to request medication cannot be restricted or stopped by contracts, wills, insurance policies, or other agreements. The Department of Human Services—Health Services requires physicians to report all prescriptions to the state. Compliance confers protection from criminal prosecution. Physicians and health care systems may choose not to participate.

11.7.8 New Mexico

Elizabeth Whitefield End of Life Options Act [48] **signed into Law** Apr. 8, 2021, **effective Date** June 18, 2021.

New Mexico Department of Health **Phone:** 800-432-2080.

Patient eligibility: As with other states, candidates must be 18 or older, residents of the state, and able to make their own decisions and communicate them. A patient must have a terminal illness with a life expectancy of 6 months or less. **Physician requirements:** The doctor must diagnose a terminal illness with a life expectancy of 6 months or less and ensure that patient is either enrolled in a hospice program, or that one other health care provider has confirmed the patient's diagnosis and 6-month life expectancy. If either doctor questions the patient's ability to make judgments, the patient must be referred for a psychological examination. Prescribing doctor confirms lack of coercion and ability to administer medication. Prescribing doctor must inform the patient of alternatives, including hospice, palliative care, and pain management options. Prescribing doctor must offer opportunity to withdraw request. **Patient request timeline:** Written request to their doctor, signed in front of two qualified, adult witnesses. Use specific form. **Other:** Patient's ability to request medication cannot be restricted or stopped by contracts, wills, insurance policies, or other agreements. Physicians and health care systems may choose not to participate.

11.7.9 Oregon

1. Ballot Measure 16**: Death With Dignity Act [49] Passed:** Nov. 8, 1994 (51% in favor), **effective Date** October 27, 1997.

2. Ballot Measure 51: **Repeals Death with Dignity Act** Passed: Nov. 4, 1997 (60% against).

3. Supreme Court of the United States: *Gonzales v. State of Oregon* Decided: Jan. 17, 2006 (6-3 in favor of the State of Oregon), upholds ***Death With Dignity Act***. Court majority opinion held that the *Controlled Substances Act* does not empower

the Attorney General of the United States to prohibit doctors from prescribing regulated drugs for use in physician-assisted suicide under state law permitting the procedure.

4. SB 579 Changes **Death with Dignity Act** [50]. Signed into law July 24, 2019, allowing patients with fewer than 15 days to live to submit the second oral request for life-ending medication at any time after the first oral request, bypassing the 15-day waiting period.

5. Mar. 29, 2022 – Oregon Ends Residency Requirement In a court settlement with Compassion & Choices, the Oregon Health Authority and the Oregon Medical Board agreed to stop enforcing the residency requirement and to ask the legislature to amend the law.

Oregon Health Authority **Phone:** 971-673-1222 **Email:** dwda.info@state.or.us

Patient eligibility: As with other states, candidates must be 18 or older, without a requirement for state residency, and able to make their own decisions and communicate them. A patient must have a terminal illness with a life expectancy of 6 months or less. **Physician requirements:** The doctor must diagnose a terminal illness with a life expectancy of 6 months or less. This must be confirmed by a second consulting doctor, who is also expected to certify that the patient can make and communicate health care decisions. If either doctor questions the patient's ability to make judgments, the patient must be referred for a psychological examination. The attending doctor must inform the patient of alternatives, including palliative care, hospice, and pain management options. The doctor must request that the patient notify next of kin. **Patient request timeline:** First oral request to physician, 15-day waiting period for patients who are expected to live more than 15 days (no waiting for patients nearer death). Second oral request to physician, written request to physician, 48-hour waiting period before picking up prescribed medications from pharmacy. **Other:** Patient's health or life insurance policies cannot be affected by use of law. The Department of Human Services—Health Services requires physicians to report all prescriptions to the state. Compliance ensures protection from criminal prosecution. Physicians and health care systems may choose not to participate.

11.7.10 Vermont

Act 39 **An Act Relating to Patient Choice and Control at End of Life [51] signed into Law** May 20, 2013 **effective Date:** May 20, 2013.

Vermont Department of Health **Phone:** 800-464-4343.

Patient eligibility: As with other states, candidates must be 18 or older, residents of the state, and able to make their own decisions and communicate them. A patient must have a terminal illness with a life expectancy of 6 months or less.

Physician requirements: The doctor must diagnose a terminal illness with a life expectancy of 6 months or less. This must be confirmed by a second consulting doctor, who is also expected to certify that the patient can make and communicate health care decisions. If either doctor questions the patient's ability to make judgments, the patient must be referred for a psychological examination. The attending doctor must inform the patient of alternatives, including palliative care, hospice, and pain management options.

Patient request timeline: First oral request to doctor, 15-day waiting period, second oral request to doctor along with written request; 48 h to dispense.

Other: Insurance policies are protected from being affected by patient's decision to use law. Physicians and health care systems may choose not to participate.

11.7.11 Washington

Ballot Initiative 1000: Death With Dignity Act [52] **voted On** Nov. 4, 2008 (58% in favor), **effective Date** March 5, 2009.

Washington State Department of Health Phone: 360-236-4030.

Patient eligibility: As with other states, candidates must be 18 or older, residents of the state, and able to make their own decisions and communicate them. A patient must have a terminal illness with a life expectancy of 6 months or less.

Physician requirements: The doctor must diagnose a terminal illness with a life expectancy of 6 months or less. This must be confirmed by a second consulting doctor, who is also expected to certify that the patient can make and communicate health care decisions. If either doctor questions the patient's ability to make judgments, the patient must be referred for a psychological examination. The attending doctor must inform the patient of alternatives, including palliative care, hospice, and pain management options. The doctor should request that the patient notify next of kin.

Patient request timeline: First oral request to doctor, 15-day waiting period, second oral request to doctor along with written request; 48 h to dispense.

Other: Patient's health or life insurance policies cannot be affected by use of law. The Department of Health requires physicians to report all prescriptions to the state. Compliance is the condition for protection from criminal prosecution. Physicians and health care systems may choose not to participate.

12. Conclusion

We set out to discuss every way a patient could deliberately shorten life in 2022. We believed that a truthful presentation of choices and the consequences that could accrue might lead a patient, after extensive reading and contemplation, to seek help with fears and suffering and make peace with living among us as long as life holds out. We made this presentation even though we have come to have increasingly grave reservations about the wisdom of allowing doctors to kill people while protected by the state.

Acknowledgements

The authors wish to acknowledge the assistance and forbearance of our spouses Kurt Berninger and Janice Plumer in creating this project.

Conflict of interest

No conflicts of interest are identified for either author.

Author details

Michael H. Plumer* and Margaret C. Cecil
Las Vegas, Nevada, USA

*Address all correspondence to: mplumer44@gmail.com

References

[1] Sulmasy LS, Mueller PS. Ethics and the legalization of physician-assisted suicide: an American College of Physicians position paper. Annals of Internal Medicine. 2021;**167**(8):576-578. DOI: 10.7326/M17-0938

[2] Oregon 2020 Report. Available from: www.oregon.gov/oha/PH/PROVIDERPARTNERRESOURCES/EVALUATIONRESEARCH/DEATHWITHDIGNITYACT/Documents/year23.pdf. [Accessed: August 5, 2022]

[3] Oregon 2021 Report. Available from: https://www.oregon.gov/oha/PH/PROVIDERPARTNERRESOURCES/EVALUATIONRESEARCH/DEATHWITHDIGNITYACT/Documents/year24.pdf. [Accessed: May 29, 2022]

[4] Hippocratic Oath. Available from: https://www.nlm.nih.gov/hmd/greek/greek_oath.html. [Accessed: August 6, 2022]

[5] Rubenfeld S, Sulmasy DP. Physician-Assisted Suicide and Euthanasia: Before, during, and after the Holocaust. Lexington, London; 2020. 344 p. ISBN 9781793609496 (cloth)

[6] Humphry D. Final Exit: The practicalities of self-deliverance and assisted suicide for the dying. New York: Dell; 2011. ISBN13 9780385336536 (paperback)

[7] Nitschke P, Stewart F. The Peaceful Pill Handbook. WA: Exit International; 2020. ISBN 9798645057718

[8] US Hospice Documents. Available from: www.cms.gov/files/document/model-hospice-election-statement-and-addendum.pdf. [Accessed: August 6, 2022]

[9] Shifting Hospice Service. Available from: https://www.nhpco.org/nhpcos-new-facts-and-figures-report-shows-changes-in-hospice-patient-diagnoses/. [Accessed: August 6, 2022]

[10] American Academy of Hospice and Palliative Medicine. Advisory Brief: Guidance on Responding to Requests for Physician-Assisted Dying. Available from: http://aahpm.org/positions/padbrief. [Accessed: August 6, 2022]

[11] Oregon 2021 Death With Dignity reference. Available from: www.oregon.gov/oha/PH/PROVIDERPARTNERRESOURCES/EVALUATIONRESEARCH/DEATHWITHDIGNITYACT/Documents/year24.pdf. [Accessed: August 6, 2022]

[12] Vizcarrondo FE. Neonatal euthanasia: The Groningen Protocol. Linacre Q. 2014;**81**(4):388-392. DOI: 10.1179/0024363914Z.00000000086. PMID: 25473136; PMCID: PMC4240050

[13] Nuland SB. How We Die. NY: Knopf; 1993. 278 p. ISBN 0-679-41461-4

[14] Värnik P. Suicide in the world. International Journal of Environmental Research and Public Health. 2012;**9**(3):760-771. DOI: 10.3390/ijerph9030760

[15] Ritchie H, Roser M, Ortiz-Ospina E. Suicide. Our World in Data. Available from: https://ourworldindata.org/suicide. [Accessed: May 5, 2022]

[16] US States Ranked by Suicide Rate. Available from: https://www.beckershospitalreview.com/rankings-and-ratings/us-states-ranked-by-suicide-rate-072121.html. [Accessed: May 29, 2022]

[17] Informed Consent SCOTUS. Available from: https://biotech.law.lsu.edu/cases/consent/cruzan_sc.htm. [Accessed: August 6, 2022]

[18] Quill TE, Menzel PT, Pope TM, Schwarz JK. Voluntarily Stopping Eating and Drinking: A Compassionate, Widely Available Option for Hastening Death. Oxford, NY; 2021. 278 p. ISBN 9780190080730 (hardback)

[19] Schwarz JK. Stopping eating and drinking. The American Journal of Nursing. 2009;**109**:53-60

[20] Bolt EE, Hagens M, Willems D, Onwuteaka-Phillipsen BD. Primary care patients hastening death by voluntarily stopping eating and drinking. Annals of Family Medicine. 2015;**13**(5):421-428. DOI: 10.1370/afm.1814. Available from: https://www.ncbi.nlm.nih.gov/pmc/articles/PMC4569449/. [Accessed: May 30, 2022]

[21] Euthanasia and Physician-Assisted Suicide (PAS) Around the World. 2021. Available from: https://www.procon.org/euthanasia-physician-assisted-suicide-pas-around-the-world/. [Accessed: March 15, 2022]

[22] Euthanasia Rates in Netherlands. Available from: https://healthcare-in-europe.com/en/news/a-critical-look-at-the-rising-euthanasia-rates-in-the-netherlands.html. [Accessed: August 6, 2022]

[23] Belgium Analysis of 2020 Commission Report. Available from: https://www.ieb-eib.org/en/news/end-of-life/euthanasia-and-assisted-suicide/euthanasia-in-belgium-analysis-of-the-2020-commission-report-1921.html. [Accessed: August 6, 2022]

[24] Luxembourg Conditions. Available from: https://guichet.public.lu/en/citoyens/famille/euthanasie-soins-palliatifs/fin-de-vie/euthanasie-assistance-suicide.html#bloub-4. [Accessed: August 6, 2022]

[25] National Commission for Control and Evaluation Suicide Rates. Available from: https://oneofus.eu/euthanasia-deaths-increase-56-in-luxembourg-in-2020/. [Accessed: August 6, 2022]

[26] Canada Bill C-14. Available from: https://www.parl.ca/DocumentViewer/en/42-1/bill/C-14/royal-assent. [Accessed: August 6, 2022]

[27] Canada MAID Eligibility. Available from: https://www.canada.ca/en/health-canada/services/medical-assistance-dying.html. [Accessed: August 6, 2022]

[28] Canada 13K Euthanasia. Available from: https://www.canada.ca/en/health-canada/services/medical-assistance-dying/annual-report-2020.html. [Accessed: August 6, 2022]

[29] Canada Bill C-7. Available from: https://parl.ca/DocumentViewer/en/43-2/bill/C-7/royal-assent. [Accessed: August 6, 2022]

[30] Canada Most Permissive. Available from: https://nationalpost.com/health/canada-mental-illness-maid-medical-aid-in-dying#:~:text=One%20year%20from%20now%2C%20in,or%20any%20other%20mental%20affliction. [Accessed: August 6, 2022]

[31] Spain. Available from: https://www.bbc.com/news/world-europe-56446631. [Accessed: August 6, 2022]

[32] Colombia. Available from: https://www.patientsrightscouncil.org/site/colombia/. [Accessed: August 6, 2022]

[33] Finland. Available from: https://stm.fi/en/-/expert-working-group-proposes-changes-to-palliative-care-no-shared-

view-on-the-legalisation-of-euthanasia. [Accessed: August 6, 2022]

[34] Germany. Available from: https://www.dw.com/en/assisted-suicide-german-government-seeks-to-regulate-practice/a-56384539. [Accessed: August 6, 2022]

[35] New Zealand. Available from: https://www.health.govt.nz/our-work/life-stages/assisted-dying-service. [Accessed: August 6, 2022]

[36] New Zealand Report. Available from: https://www.health.govt.nz/our-work/life-stages/assisted-dying-service/assisted-dying-service-data-and-reporting. [Accessed: August 6, 2022]

[37] Switzerland. Available from: http://www.dignitas.ch/index.php?option=com_content&view=article&id=22&Itemid=5&lang=en. [Accessed: August 5, 2022]

[38] Bloom A. In Love: A Memoir of Love and Loss. NY: Random House; 2022. 210 p. ISBN 9780593243947 (hardcover)

[39] Amy Bloom. Available from: https://www.npr.org/sections/health-shots/2022/03/08/1084912553/alzheimers-assisted-suicide-amy-bloom-in-love. [Accessed: August 6, 2022]

[40] State by State Physician-Assisted Suicide Statistics. 2019. Available from: https://www.procon.org/state-by-state-physician-assisted-suicide-statistics/. [Accessed: August 6, 2022]

[41] CA ABX2-12 End of Life Option Act. Available from: https://images.procon.org/wp-content/uploads/sites/43/end-of-life-option-act-ca.pdf. [Accessed: August 6, 2022]

[42] CO Proposition 106 End of Life Options Act. Available from: https://efaidnbmnnnibpcajpcglclefindmkaj/https://images.procon.org/wp-content/uploads/sites/43/colorado-physician-assisted-suicide-law-2016.pdf. [Accessed: August 6, 2022]

[43] DC 21-577 Death With Dignity Act of 2016. Available from: https://images.procon.org/wp-content/uploads/sites/43/dc-signed-law.pdf. [Accessed: August 6, 2022]

[44] Hawai'i HB 2739 Our Care our Choice Act. Available from: https://images.procon.org/wp-content/uploads/sites/43/hawaii-pas-legalization.pdf. [Accessed: August 6, 2022]

[45] ME HP 948, An Act to Enact the Maine Death With Dignity Act. Available from: https://www.mainelegislature.org/legis/bills/bills_129th/billtexts/HP094801.asp. [Accessed: August 6, 2022]

[46] MT First Judicial District Court Baxter vs Montana. Available from: https://images.procon.org/wp-content/uploads/sites/43/mccarter_opinion_montana.pdf. [Accessed: August 6, 2022]

[47] NJ A1504 Aid in Dying for the Terminally Ill Act. Available from: https://images.procon.org/wp-content/uploads/sites/43/new-jersey-pas-law-a1504.pdf. [Accessed: August 6, 2022]

[48] NM Elizabeth Whitefield End of Life Options Act. Available from: https://www.nmlegis.gov/Sessions/21%20Regular/bills/house/HB0047.pdf. [Accessed: August 6, 2022]

[49] OR Ballot Measure 16 Death With Dignity Act. Available from: https://images.procon.org/wp-content/uploads/sites/43/ordeathwithdignityact.pdf. [Accessed: August 5, 2022]

[50] SB 579 Changes Death With Dignity Act. Available from: https://images.procon.org/wp-content/uploads/sites/43/oregon-sb-579-2019.pdf. [Accessed: August 5, 2022]

[51] Vermont Act 39 An act Relating to Patient Choice and Control at End of Life. Available from: https://images.procon.org/wp-content/uploads/sites/43/act039_vermont_death_with_dignity.pdf. [Accessed: August 6, 2022]

[52] WA Ballot Initiative 10000: Death With Dignity Act. Available from: https://images.procon.org/wp-content/uploads/sites/43/euthwashingtonstatelaw.pdf. [Accessed: August 6, 2022]

Chapter 11

Prognostic Communication in the Era of Targeted Therapy and Immunotherapy

Sherri Cervantez, Matthew Butler and Anand Karnad

Abstract

Effectively communicating prognosis to patients with cancer is a key communication task for physicians. It has always been a difficult task and is now becoming more so. Rapid progress in treatment of advanced cancers is transforming a previously terminal illness with its proverbial <6 months of life expectancy into a chronic illness with years of meaningful quality of life ahead. Despite this evolution, the importance of communicating prognosis to enable shared decision-making cannot change. Communication skills for this specific task should be strengthened and refined with practice and toolkits to enable physicians to rise to the unique challenge of discussing prognosis in this rapidly shifting milieu of cancer care. This chapter will first discuss how targeted and immunotherapy have changed the landscape of cancer therapy and complicated prognostication through representative case examples. Secondly, we will outline communication preferences, barriers to prognostication, and tools useful in cancer prognostication. Finally, we will identify techniques palliative physicians and oncologists utilize to convey prognostic information vital to patient decision-making.

Keywords: prognostication, communication, immunotherapy, targeted therapy, cancer therapy

1. Introduction

For a patient with cancer, prognosis, the prediction, or estimation of the likely course, has profound effects: preparing to face mortality, making decisions regarding treatments, and hoping for ideal outcomes for the future. Communicating prognosis is central to shared decision-making and autonomy [1, 2], and understanding prognostic information can influence patients' decisions on whether to receive life extending care [3, 4]. Poor communication therefore can lead to poor outcomes.

Prognostic disclosure in oncology care has been shown to be an essential component of good clinical practice for children [5], adolescent and young adults [6] and on up to the very elderly [7]. Despite the acknowledged importance of communicating prognosis in cancer care, this task has remained a challenge with multiple barriers: physician discomfort in discussing prognosis, patient diversity and other barriers to receiving prognostic information, and patient's family raising barriers of their own in their belief and acceptance of prognosis. Oncologist's skills and experiences and comfort level in managing patients' reactions to prognostic information has emerged as a principal barrier to high-quality prognostic communication [8]. Adding to all these factors are the significant challenges brought about by the rapid advances bringing an array of new and effective treatment for many advanced cancers.

This review will briefly discuss communicating prognosis in the era of progress in cancer treatment ushered in by the identification of molecular targets leading to effective targeted therapy, and the control of advanced cancers by checkpoint inhibitors and immunotherapy. Brief discussion of patient examples to highlight the current profound complexity of discussing prognosis will help appreciate the impact of changes brought about by newer therapy on this communication task. We will provide an overview of prognostic communication preferences and barriers. We will conclude with a discussion of helpful tools and techniques to enable effective prognostic conversation.

2. Evolving landscape of cancer therapy

2.1 Effect of the progress in cancer therapy on communicating prognosis

Oncologists in training 40 years ago very easily saw the natural history of most adult cancers during the 2 or 3 years of their fellowship program. There were very few effective treatments for the most common advanced stage cancers. In that period, discussing prognosis with patients who had advanced cancer caused emotional distress in oncologists and their patients and this was a significant barrier to effective conversation about prognosis. Contrast that with what the current trainee faces in this era of targeted and immunotherapy: 50 or more new drugs for cancer treatment have been approved in both 2020 and 2021 [9, 10] and a significant decrease is now evident in cancer mortality [11] contributing to an increased lifespan [12]. Therefore, advanced cancers now are not always rapidly fatal and decision-making regarding treatment forces even the expert hematology and medical oncology physicians to pause before rendering prognostic opinions. The pause is not only to assess the impact of performance status and co-morbidities on prognosis, but also to: 1) ponder and choose from a bewildering array of treatment choices; 2) to consider the likelihood of rapid response and degree of complete remissions possible in the "exceptional responders;" 3) to consider the quality of life of patients who may have to learn to live with their cancer on maintenance therapy; and 4) to consider if the patient they face now will one day be monitored for treatment-free remissions. All these points deeply influence how we should think about discussing prognosis in patients with advanced cancer.

2.2 Prognostic communication in patients with solid tumors—Case-based discussion

2.2.1 Case #1: ALK mutated lung cancer

Take for example, a 53-year-old female with diabetes who reported a dry non-productive cough starting in March of 2017. She was evaluated by her primary care physician and found to have a mass of her right lung. Inadequate health insurance resulted in delays and a biopsy was obtained only in August 2017 confirming poorly differentiated high-grade neuroendocrine carcinoma with metastatic disease to the lumbar spine. She received palliative radiation to the spine, then started on standard systemic chemotherapy with cisplatin and etoposide but progressed after three cycles. She was then switched to standard second line immunotherapy in November. Restaging scans after three cycles revealed mixed response. At this point she was following the typical natural course of lung cancer, and without new effective therapy her prognosis would have been grim. However, molecular profiling of her tumor demonstrated an ALK mutation. She was transitioned to the targeted agent ceritinib, and experienced a near complete response (**Figure 1**). She has remained on therapy without adverse events and no evidence of disease to date far exceeding the prognostic predictions at the time of second line therapy.

2.2.2 Case #2: Metastatic non-small cell lung cancer

Consider a 64-year-old female with adenocarcinoma of the lung with metastatic disease to the retroperitoneum and pancreatic tail who was treated on a clinical trial with induction chemotherapy of carboplatin, paclitaxel, bevacizumab and atezolizumab resulting in rapid and dramatic response; followed by Atezolizumab maintenance with continued control of disease when she developed an encephalopathy syndrome due to the atezolizumab and treatment was discontinued. Off therapy, she developed rapid onset of progressive metastatic disease to bone causing large destructive lesions of her left hemipelvis requiring orthopedic surgery to stabilize her hip. She then completed radiation therapy to the involved area and then began maintenance doses of mono-immunotherapy with nivolumab without recurrence of encephalopathy. She has remained on maintenance immunotherapy for greater than 5 years with no evidence of disease enjoying an excellent quality of life with near normal performance status.

2.3 Prognostic communication in patients with hematologic malignancies—Case-based discussion

Prognostic information has generally been better studied in patients with solid tumors. Patients with hematological malignancies faced uncertain illness trajectory, treatment choices associated with risk of severe toxicity, but also a persistent chance for cure from stem cell transplant or CAR T cell therapy for the select few eligible for such options [13, 14]. Targeted therapy and immunotherapy have dramatically improved outcomes for patients with hematological malignancies [15].

2.3.1 Case #1: Multiple myeloma

A healthy man presented at age 68 with new-onset mid back pain. Imaging showed a deformity at T8 arising from a lytic lesion, along with lesions in other bones. Bone marrow biopsy demonstrated 40% clonal plasma cells, with FISH showing translocation (11, 14). Treatment was initiated with bortezomib, lenalidomide, and dexamethasone. After 2 cycles he developed grade 2 peripheral neuropathy, and bortezomib was discontinued. After 5 additional cycles of lenalidomide and dexamethasone, the monoclonal protein dropped more than 90% relative to pre-treatment baseline, meeting criteria for a very good partial response. He then received an autologous stem cell transplant, which he tolerated without major complications. Post-transplant, the monoclonal protein was undetectable, and lenalidomide maintenance was initiated. After just over two years of maintenance therapy he began to complain of worsening back pain. Imaging showed enlargement of several bony lesions with a new compression deformity at L1. His performance status remained excellent.

This example illustrates a common clinical situation of symptomatic relapse of multiple myeloma after stem cell transplant. Prior to 2012, the options for such a

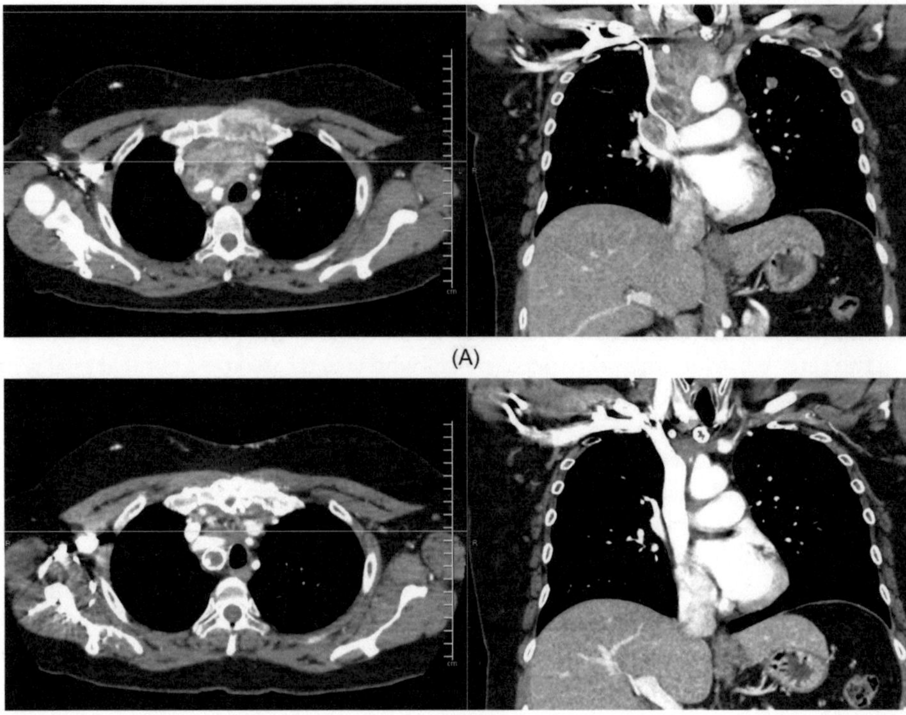

Figure 1.
A. Representative axial and coronal cross sectionals pretreatment with Alk inhibitor. B. Representative axial and coronal cross sectionals posttreatment with Alk inhibitor demonstrating near complete response.

patient would have been limited. In 2022, the array of options in the same clinical situation is broad. Pomalidomide, carfilzomib, and daratumumab are all widely used drugs offering high response rates, alone and in numerous combinations, and all have mild toxicity profiles. These drugs can be combined to make several lines of therapy, even in patients with less-than-optimal organ function and performance status. Even after a patient becomes refractory to these drugs, newer salvage options are available, including selinexor, belantamab mafodotin, and elotuzumab. Several investigational drugs are in advanced stages of development and will likely add more treatment options in the near future. CAR-T therapy is commercially available as of 2021, and offers very high response rates, while incurring high cost and complexity of treatment. Finally, the patient's 11;14 translocation makes him a candidate to receive venetoclax, which has shown activity in this subgroup. With access to these treatments, survival for five years or longer after a first relapse is becoming routine. However, the likelihood of achieving response and the duration of response tend to drop with each successive line of therapy. It is rare to exhaust all available lines of therapy, but the tradeoffs between burdens and benefits of treatment shift progressively though the course of disease.

2.3.2 Case #2: Acute myeloid leukemia

A 73-year-old woman with diabetes, hypertension, stage IV chronic kidney disease, and mild dementia presented with nausea, vomiting, and chest pain.

Laboratory tests on admission showed leukocytosis of 22,000/μL along with moderate anemia and thrombocytopenia. Bone marrow biopsy was diagnostic for acute myeloid leukemia (AML).

Management of AML in the elderly is a longstanding challenge as the benefits of intensive chemotherapy are outweighed by the risk of infections and other complications. Historically these patients were treated with lower-intensity cytotoxic regimens, which could prolong survival by a few months at best.

Hypomethylating agents (azacitidine and decitabine) in combination with the BCL-2 inhibitor venetoclax have transformed the care of the elderly AML patient giving them a median survival of 14.7 months [16]. Although the combination can be tolerated by frail elders, it is not free from toxicity. The patient described above, despite kidney disease, early dementia, and limited functional status, has no absolute contraindications to such treatment, though these factors may negatively affect tolerability. Deciding whether to start combination therapy, a single agent, or best supportive care is therefore a complex and individualized decision.

2.4 Effect of the progress in cancer therapy on clinical practice

These cases serve to illustrate the high level of complexity that exists from response to later lines of therapy, to associated toxicities, to anticipated quality of life on treatment. Targeted and immunotherapies are associated with both palliative benefits in terms of pain/symptom control and improved survival benefits compared to former cytotoxic chemotherapy options (**Table 1**). Additionally, these therapeutics are associated with fewer and less severe toxicities such that patients can remain on treatment for extended periods of time.

These factors in combination with the hope for durable responses have resulted in a shift in referral patterns for patients with advanced and metastatic disease. In a 2019 study, a trend toward fewer hospice referrals and increased subacute rehab referrals from inpatient oncology units was noted with nearly two-thirds of patients never receiving additional cancer therapy [27]. In another retrospective study of deceased patients who had received immunotherapy, two-thirds had received immunotherapy in the last 90 days of life [28]. Notably, patients who had received immunotherapy in the last 30 days of life received less than 3 doses, had a poor performance status, had lower hospice enrollment, and higher rates of dying in the hospital [28]. Although extraordinary and durable responses are seen, these two studies emphasis the prognostic dilemma, as the majority of patients are likely to follow a different natural course. Therefore, assessing patient preferences for information sharing and goals of care is essential.

3. Prognostic communication preferences in oncology

3.1 Prognostic communication clinician factors

Communication is a specialized skill. Indeed a review of the literature of prognosis related communication in advanced cancer patients suggests that it is useful to divide oncologists into three groups with respect to their ability to engage in meaningful high-quality communication with their patients: Highly skilled oncologists need organizational support and can serve as mentors; moderately skilled oncologists may benefit from

Disease	Treatment options in 2010	Prognosis circa 2010	Major developments	Prognosis in 2022
Metastatic NSCLC	Doublet or triplet cytotoxic chemotherapy	mOS approximately 10–12 months [17, 18], 5-year survival 8% [19]	EGFR agents	Targeted Therapy mOS (mo) [20]: EGFR 18–38 [21, 22]
			ALK agents	ALK 47-not reached
			ROS1	ROS1 24-not reached
			BRAF	BRAF 17
			RET	KRAS 12.5
			MET	RET, MET,NTRK data immature
			NTRK	Targeted Therapy: 5-year survival 83% [23]
			KRAS immunotherapy	Immunotherapy: Median OS 22 months (treatment naïve), 5 year survival 23% [24]
AML (older and less fit patients, not fit for intensive chemotherapy)	Low-dose cytotoxic chemotherapy	Median OS <6 months; 1-year survival 28% [25]	Hypomethylating agents, BCL-2 inhibitor	Median OS 15 months; 2-year survival 74% [16]
Multiple myeloma	Lenalidomide or bortezomib, combined with steroids and/or chemotherapy	Overall survival 1–2 years [26]	Multidrug combinations including: 2nd generation immunomodulatory drugs	OS unknown, but likely 5 years or more
			2nd generation proteosome inhibitors	
			monoclonal antibodies	
			CAR-T cellular therapy	

Table 1.
Evolution of prognosis in representative case examples.

targeted skills training; and lower skilled oncologists may benefit from pairing with high level communicators or utilization of supportive programs to facilitate effective communication [8]. Discussing prognosis does include asking patients if they wish to receive this information and being prepared to respect their decision and re-engage periodically.

DOI: http://dx.doi.org/10.5772/intechopen.105144

Communication training and skills are common barriers reported by clinicians. Inadequate training can result in brief, vague, or total avoidance of prognostic discussions. Conversely, physicians may use jargoned language with the intent to deliver accurate information or the uncertainty of prognosis, however no additional clarity is provided to the patient. Additionally, these conversations may be viewed as time consuming in the context of a busy oncology practice.

The emotional nature of prognosis contributes to additional clinician discomfort with delivering bad news and managing patient responses. Despite data suggesting otherwise, many physicians feel prognostic conversations decrease patient hope and create a less favorable provider-patient relationship [8, 29]. This poses a significant barrier as many oncologists develop a personal bond with their patients.

Finally, physician experience plays a significant role. Rapid progress in treatment has led to the finding that hematologic oncologists with fewer years of practice are less likely to engage in prognostic discussion [30] compared with younger physicians caring for patients with solid tumors who were significantly more likely to discuss prognosis than their older colleagues [31]. This reflects a higher level of "information uncertainty" and less confidence among junior hematologic oncologists as a major prognostication challenge for hematological malignancies [30].

3.2 Prognostic communication patient preferences

For patients and families, having prognostic information influences treatment preferences, decreases uncertainty and helps them to plan ahead for both personal and healthcare matters [32]. The majority of patients prefer to have prognosis communicated and nearly universally, they want accurate and honest information [33]. While some variation in preferences is influenced by age and sex, underlying cancer type and treatment goals do not impact patient preference [29]. In this era then, communication of prognosis with the elderly person with advanced cancer deserves special mention: Communicating prognosis in the elderly, especially in the very elderly (>85), or frail elderly is important for establishing patient centered goals of care and advance care planning. Fear, grief, and anxiety are common factors contributing to patient related barriers in prognostic communication and therefore invoking a patient's preference for information sharing remains essential [29]. Additionally, language and education barriers contribute to prognostic misunderstandings [29].

3.3 Impact of care giver preferences on prognostic communication

While important on an individual level, cultural and community factors often guide care giver communication preferences. For instance, South American and Asian cultures are less likely to believe patients should be told about a terminal prognosis [29]. This discrepancy between patient and family preferences can contribute to prognostic communication barriers. Discussing prognosis often involves a family member as the patient may rely increasingly on a family member for decision making and care—and the patient, especially if elderly, is often more receptive than the family when hearing prognostic information.

4. Prognostic tools

4.1 Clinician prediction of survival (CPS)

Clinician prediction of survival (CPS) is a quick and convenient estimate of survival based on clinical experience and intuition. While CPS is convenient, it is inaccurate and subject to biases with consistent over estimation of survival. Literature review suggests CPS is accurate 20–30% of the time with ~80% of prognostic errors being overoptimistic [33]. Overestimation may lead to overtreatment and delayed referrals to palliative care. Conversely, while less common, underestimation can result in undertreatment and premature referral to hospice or supportive services [33]. CPS can be classified by several approaches. The most common technique utilized by clinicians is a temporal approach which attempts to answer "How long will the patient live?" or providing an estimated duration of survival [32]. A probabilistic approach estimates "What is the probability of survival in a specific time frame?" (i.e. 30% chance of being alive in 6 months) [32]. Alternatively, the surprise question is utilized to determine "Would I be surprised if a patient died in the next year?" [34]. The surprise question significantly improves clinician accuracy in predicting poor prognosis. In order to provide the most accurate prognosis several models have been developed to facilitate clinical communication. While these validated models provide more objective prognosis, they do not necessarily capture the nuances of an individual's health.

4.2 Palliative prognostic score (PaP)

The palliative prognostic score was initially developed in Italy to be used as an estimate of short-term survival [35, 36]. PaP combines CPS, Karofsky Performance Score (KPS) and five clinical/laboratory variables including performance status, dyspnea, anorexia, leukocyte count, lymphocyte percentage (**Figure 2**) [37]. Each criterion is assigned a score which are then summed to generate a numerical score (0–17.5). The values are then stratified into three groups according to a 30-day survival probability. The PaP has been validated in advanced cancer settings and shown to be accurate irrespective of cancer type [38]. In an interesting validation study, the inclusion of CPS as a criterion enhanced the accuracy [39].

4.3 Palliative performance scale (PPS)

The PPS, originally developed in 1996, is a reliable, validated tool which uses five observer-rated domains correlated to the Karnofsky Performance Scale (100–0%) with scores in 10% decrements (**Figure 3**) [40–42]. The domains include ambulation, activity level/evidence of disease, self-care, intake, and level of consciousness. PPS scores are determined based on a "best fit" while reading downward through a single domain and then across the remaining domains left to right. If several domains are categorized at one level and other domains at a higher or lower level, clinical judgement and leftward precedence is used to determine the more accurate score. While the PPS may be used for different purposes, it is a key tool for quickly communicating a patient's functional level. More importantly, the PPS is a valuable prognostic tool as scores correlate with actual survival and median survival time for cancer patients in the ambulatory setting thereby allowing estimates in terms of days, weeks, months, and years (**Figure 4**) [43, 44].

Characteristic	PaP Partial Score
Dypnea	
No	0
Yes	1.0
Anorexia	
No	0
Yes	1.5
Karnofsky performance status	
≥50	0
30–40	0
10–20	2.5
Clinical prediction of survival (weeks)	
>12	0
11–12	2.0
9–10	2.5
7–8	2.5
5–6	4.5
3–4	6.0
1–2	8.5
Total white blood count (cell/mm^3)	
Normal (4800–8500)	0
High (8501–11000)	0.5
Very high (>11000)	1.5
Lymphocyte rate (%)	
Normal (20.0–40.0)	0
Low (12.0–19.9)	1.0
Very low (0–11.9)	2.5
Risk groups	**PaP Total score**
A (30-day survival probability >70%)	0.0–5.5
B (30-day survival probability 30–70%)	5.6–11.0
C (30-day survival probability <30%)	11.1–17.5

Total scores range between 0 and 17.5, and patients were assigned to one of three different risk groups according to a 30-day survival probability: group A, <70%; group B, 30–70%; and group C, >30%.

Figure 2.
Palliative prognostic score.

4.4 Palliative prognostic index

The Palliative Prognostic Index(PPI) was originally developed in Japan for hospice in patients with advanced cancer [45]. PPI utilizes PPS, oral intake, and the presence or absence of dyspnea, edema, and delirium (**Figure 5**) [46]. Criteria are assigned a numeric score and the total is stratified into one of three groups, predicting survival of shorter than three weeks (PPI score greater than 6), shorter than six weeks (PPI score greater than 4), or more than six weeks (PPI score less than or equal to 4) [47].

4.5 Terminal cancer prognostic index

The Terminal Cancer Prognostic score (TCP score) is based on the weighted scores of three predictors (diarrhea, anorexia, and confusion), which were determined in multivariate analysis to be independent predictors of survival for terminally ill cancer patients (**Figure 6**) [46, 48]. The scores are then used to differentiate into

PPS Level	Ambulation	Activity & Evidence of Disease	Self-Care	Intake	Conscious Level
100%	Full	Normal activity & work No evidence of disease	Full	Normal	Full
90%	Full	Normal activity & work Some evidence of disease	Full	Normal	Full
80%	Full	Normal activity with Effort Some evidence of disease	Full	Normal or reduced	Full
70%	Reduced	Unable Normal Job/Work Significant disease	Full	Normal or reduced	Full
60%	Reduced	Unable hobby/house work Significant disease	Occasional assistance necessary	Normal or reduced	Full or confusion
50%	Mainly Sit/Lie	Unable to do any work Extensive disease	Considerable assistance required	Normal or reduced	Full or confusion
40%	Mainly in bed	Unable to do most activity Extensive disease	Mainly assistance	Normal or reduced	Full or drowsy +/- confusion
30%	Totally Bed bound	Unable to do any activity Extensive disease	Total Care	Normal or reduced	Full or drowsy +/- confusion
20%	Totally Bed bound	Unable to do any activity Extensive disease	Total Care	Minimal to sips	Full or drowsy +/- confusion
10%	Totally Bed bound	Unable to do any activity Extensive disease	Total Care	Mouth care only	Drowsy or coma +/- confusion
0%	Death	-	-	-	-

Figure 3.
Palliative performance scale version 2 (PPSv2).

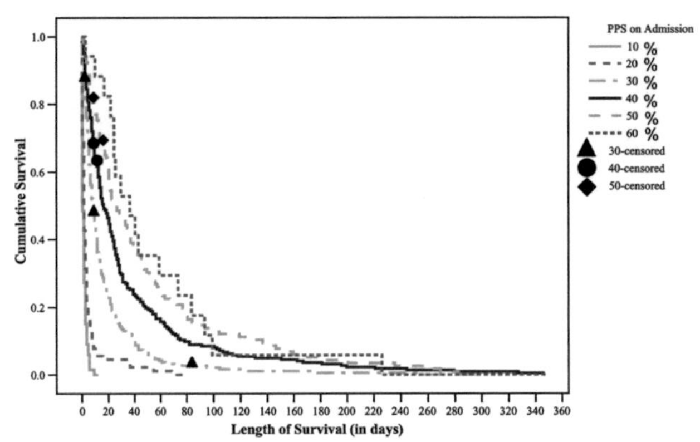

Figure 4.
Survival curves of cases with different PPS.

a prognostic group. While developed in a prospective study, this tool has not been adequately validated and is not as commonly utilized [46].

4.6 Poor prognostic indicator

In a similar pattern to the TCP score, the poor prognostic indicator is a score developed based on dysphagia, cognitive failure, and weight loss in the last 6 months [46, 49]. The score has a PPV of 0.76 at estimating 4-week mortality for patients with advanced cancer admitted to a palliative care unit. This prospective study demonstrated that the poor prognostic indicator was as effective in predictions of survival as two skilled physicians, although this tool has also not been adequately validated [49].

Variable		Partial score value
Palliative performance scale (modified Karnofsky)		
10–20		4
30–50		2.5
≥60		0
Oral intake		
Severely reduced		2.5
Moderately reduced		1.0
Normal		0
Oedema		
Present		1.0
Absent		0.0
Dyspnoea at rest		
Present		3.5
Absent		0.0
Delirium		
Present		4.0
Absent		0.0
Interpretation of the PPI score		
Total score	PPV for 6-week survival	NPV for 6-week survival
>4	0.83	0.71

PPV, positive predictive value; NPV, negative predictive value.

Figure 5.
Palliative prognostic index.

4.7 Charlson comorbidity index (CCI)

First developed in 1987 as a weighted approach to assess risk of death within 1-year of hospitalization with specific comorbid conditions [50]. The index assigns value to 19 medical conditions (i.e., diabetes, heart failure, peripheral vascular disease, chronic pulmonary disease, liver disease, renal disease, hemiplegia, etc.) according to presence and severity. The sum is used to estimate the risk of death. CCI is the most common comorbidity assessment utilized and has been validated in multiple solid and hematologic malignancies [51–54].

4.8 Prognostic tools in clinical practice

As mentioned, CPS is the most used method; however, the accuracy is bolstered significantly when used in combination with other more objective tools. The PaP likely has the greatest potential utility however it is unclear why this tool is not used more universally other than lack of familiarity. PPS and CCI are the most broadly used tools in both oncology and palliative care settings and have the most robust data in terms of validity in patients with cancer. Both tools also assist with longer

	Severity	Partial score
Diarrhoea		
None to mild	0–1	0
Moderate to severe	2–3	3
Anorexia		
None to mild	0–1	0
Moderate to severe	2–3	2
Confusion		
None	0	0
Mild, moderate or severe	1–3	2
Interpretation of the TCP		
Total score	Median survival time (days)	
0	103	
2	46	
4	28	
>4	25.5	

Figure 6.
Terminal cancer prognostic index.

term prognostication which is increasingly important as cancer care transitions from anticipated acute mortality to a chronic illness with associated morbidity and mortality.

5. Prognostic communication techniques

While developing and communicating prognosis is critical for patient care, evidence-based recommendations for these processes are limited. In 2005, a Working Group of the Research Network of the European Association for Palliative Care found that prognostication is feasible with the use of certain clinical tools [55]. The working group found the strongest evidence of prognostic correlation with the use of clinical prediction of survival in conjunction with performance status, symptoms associated with cancer anorexia-cachexia syndrome (weight loss, anorexia, dysphagia, and xerostomia), dyspnea, delirium, and some biologic factors (leukocytosis, lymphocytopenia, and C-reactive protein) [55]. More recently in an opinion statement, similar factors were identified as key to more accurate prognostication [56]. In addition to using validated prognostic tools to complement clinical judgement, the authors recommended seeking multi-professional prognostic estimates, formulating and recording prognosis estimates in order to better cultivate prognostic skill, and receiving training in advanced communication skills to better deliver prognostic conversations [56].

Every cancer is a complex clinical phenomenon, whose outcome is influenced by many variables: the age, underlying health, and motivation of the patient; their social support system; the availability of advanced treatments, clinicians' ability to choose and manage these treatments, patient's ability to access and afford these treatments and tolerate their side effects; and critically, the biology of the cancer itself. Even in an age of molecular and genetic tumor profiling and validated prognostic models, an estimate of prognosis is an educated guess. Clinicians must make this guess in the most accurate and objective way possible, and then use communication techniques that effectively convey the information to the patient and caregivers, while being sensitive to their receptiveness and ability to process this information.

Surveys have consistently shown that majorities of patients prefer to receive accurate and honest prognostic information, [33, 57] including average and best-case survival outcomes [58]. However, this is not universal: there is considerable variation in how much prognostic information patients and caregivers wish to receive [13, 59]. This can change over the course of illness: as the disease becomes more advanced, the patient may want less detailed prognostic information, while caregivers may need more. Therefore, prognostic discussion calls for an individualized approach, which elicits permission from patients and caregivers to discuss prognosis, and uses explicit questions and implicit cues to determine how much prognostic information to impart [3, 60, 61]. Information needs and preferences should be reassessed any time there is a significant change in the condition, prognosis, or living circumstances of the patient.

An effective discussion of prognosis is not limited to a prediction of medical outcomes, but should integrate affective communication including expressions of support and empathy, demonstration of expertise, reassurance of non-abandonment, and reinforcement of a collaborative relationship [60, 62]. Assuming permission has been given to offer predictions regarding outcome, it is important to utilize the opportunity to openly and directly discuss prognosis [61]. Clinicians should be as transparent as possible about the basis for the estimate – multiple studies, a single clinical trial, or simply an estimate based on personal clinical experience – and about the associated uncertainties.

Presenting a range of possible outcomes is a useful technique to convey the scope of uncertainty, and is preferred by patients over more narrow predictions [63]. Effort should be taken to counteract the tendency of both clinicians and patients to focus on the most favorable potential outcome. One way to frame this is surprise: describing a relatively favorable outcome but stating that it would be surprising, implying that it should not be assumed. The surprising outcome can then be contrasted against other outcomes which are expected or feared. This is one form of the best case/worst case framework, which invites hope for a favorable outcome, while encouraging preparation for a more adverse one. This approach was first studied in the context of high-risk surgery, [64, 65] but it is broadly applicable in any situation where plausible outcome scenarios differ widely. In addition to best and worst, a third scenario for the typical or average case, but it is important to emphasize that this is not a prediction, and that the best and worst outcomes remain possible.

There is no one-size-fits-all approach to improving communication skills. For delivering prognostic information, collaboration with other cancer clinicians, oncology nurses, and palliative care specialists is encouraged [66]. REMAP (Reframe, Expect emotions, Map out patient goals, Align with goals, and Propose a plan) has been suggested as a framework for goals of care conversations [67].

Indeed viewing communication interactions from a procedural lens (procedures require specialized skills, have component steps, are intentional in purpose, and have pause points and a known set of complications) may improve quality of prognostic communication [68]. In discussing the use of prognostic tools in communicating prognosis, it is useful to quote from a paper by Lakin et al., entitled, Timeout Before Talking: Communication as a medical procedure: "Skilled communication requires nuance, adjustments, and careful thought, in complex interpersonal interactions. Just as surgery is a technical intervention and a practiced art form, communication procedures require both thoughtful structure and flexible skill. When a communication task is deconstructed, it can be better applied, taught, legislated, and researched, ultimately allowing for iterative improvement of this foundational medical practice" [68].

6. Conclusions

Prognostication is an evolving science. As newer therapeutics extend and improve the expectations of critical illness management, transparency and accuracy are key factors of value to patients. For clinicians, continuing education in communication and routinely rehearsing difficult conversations may promote easier and more transparent conversations. Utilization of prognostic tools in combination with clinician prediction and interdisciplinary consensus improves overall accuracy in uncertain circumstances. Prognostic discussions should be viewed by the clinician and patient as fluid. Routinely re-evaluating and modifying prognostic estimates based on current individual circumstances, changing health status, and therapeutic advances are critical to support patient centered decision making.

Conflict of interest

The authors declare no conflict of interest.

Notes/thanks/other declarations

Figures 2, 5, and **6** reprinted from Stone PC, Lund S. Predicting prognosis in patients with advanced cancer. Annals of Oncology. 2007;18(6):971-976, with permission from Elsevier.

Figure 3 reprinted with permission from ©Victoria Hospice Society, Canada. www.victoriahospice.org.

Figure 4 reprinted from Morita T, Tsunoda J, Inoue S, Chihara S. Validity of the palliative performance scale from a survival perspective. Journal of Pain and Symptom Management. 1999;18(1):2-3, with permission from Elsevier.

Author details

Sherri Cervantez*, Matthew Butler and Anand Karnad
UT Health San Antonio MD Anderson Mays Cancer Center, Long School of Medicine, San Antonio, USA

*Address all correspondence to: cervantezs@uthscsa.edu

References

[1] LeBlanc TW, Marron JM, Ganai S, McGinnis MM, Spence RA, Tenner L, et al. Prognostication and communication in oncology. Journal of Oncology Practice/ American Society of Clinical Oncology. 2019;**15**(4):208-215

[2] Elwyn G, Frosch D, Thomson R, Joseph-Williams N, Lloyd A, Kinnersley P, et al. Shared decision making: A model for clinical practice. Journal of General Internal Medicine. 2012;**27**(10):1361-1367

[3] Mack JW, Weeks JC, Wright AA, Block SD, Prigerson HG. End-of-life discussions, goal attainment, and distress at the end of life: Predictors and outcomes of receipt of care consistent with preferences. Journal of Clinical Oncology: Official Journal of the American Society of Clinical Oncology. 2010;**28**(7):1203-1208

[4] Weeks JC, Cook EF, O'Day SJ, Peterson LM, Wenger N, Reding D, et al. Relationship between cancer patients' predictions of prognosis and their treatment preferences. Journal of the American Medical Association. 1998;**279**(21):1709-1714

[5] Sisk BA, Schulz G. Moving toward a basic science of prognostic communication. Pediatrics. 2021;**147**(6):e2021050208

[6] Mack JW, Fasciano KM, Block SD. Communication about prognosis with adolescent and young adult patients with cancer: Information needs, prognostic awareness, and outcomes of disclosure. Journal of Clinical Oncology: Official Journal of the American Society of Clinical Oncology. 2018;**36**(18):1861-1867

[7] Smith AK, Williams BA, Lo B. Discussing overall prognosis with the very elderly. The New England Journal of Medicine. 2011;**365**(23):2149-2151

[8] Al-Issa K, Helft PR. Narrative review of prognosis related communication in advanced cancer patients. Annals of Palliative Medicine. 2021;**10**(8):9239-9250

[9] Olivier T, Haslam A, Prasad V. Anticancer drugs approved by the US Food and Drug Administration From 2009 to 2020 According to Their Mechanism of Action. JAMA Network Open. 2021;**4**(12):e2138793

[10] Mullard A. 2021 FDA approvals. Nature Reviews: Drug Discovery. 2022;**21**(2):83-88

[11] Siegel RL, Miller KD, Fuchs HE, Jemal A. Cancer Statistics, 2021. CA: A Cancer Journal for Clinicians. 2021;**71**(1):7-33

[12] Products - Data Briefs - Number 427 - December 2021 [Internet]. 2021 [cited 2022 Apr 10]. Available from: https://www.cdc.gov/nchs/products/databriefs/db427.htm

[13] Gray TF, Temel JS, El-Jawahri A. Illness and prognostic understanding in patients with hematologic malignancies. Blood Reviews. 2021;**45**:100692

[14] Goldsmith SR, Ghobadi A, Dipersio JF. Hematopoeitic cell transplantation and CAR T-cell therapy: Complements or competitors? Frontiers in Oncology. 2020;**30**:10

[15] Shahid K, Khalife M, Dabney R, Phan AT. Immunotherapy and targeted

therapy—The new roadmap in cancer treatment. Annals of Translational Medicine. 2019;**7**(20):595-595

[16] DiNardo CD, Jonas BA, Pullarkat V, Thirman MJ, Garcia JS, Wei AH, et al. Azacitidine and Venetoclax in previously untreated acute myeloid leukemia. The New England Journal of Medicine. 2020;**383**(7):617-629

[17] Bagley SJ, Mitra N, Meropol NJ, Holzman B, Cohen RB, Langer CJ, et al. Comparative effectiveness of carboplatin-pemetrexed (Carbo-Pem) with vs. without bevacizumab (Bev) in patients with advanced non-squamous (Sq) non-small cell lung cancer (NSCLC). Journal of Clinical Oncology. 2018;**36**(15):9073

[18] Socinski MA, Patel JD, Garon EB, Govindan R, Reynolds CH, Spigel DR, et al. A phase III study of pemetrexed (Pem) plus carboplatin (Cb) plus bevacizumab (Bev) followed by maintenance pem plus bev versus paclitaxel (Pac) plus cb plus bev followed by maintenance bev in stage IIIb or IV nonsquamous non-small cell lung cancer (NS-NSCLC): Overall and age group results. Journal of Clinical Oncology. 2013;**31**(15):8004

[19] Lung Cancer Survival Rates | 5-Year Survival Rates for Lung Cancer. 2022. Available from: https://www.cancer.org/cancer/lung-cancer/detection-diagnosis-staging/survival-rates.html

[20] Majeed U, Manochakian R, Zhao Y, Lou Y. Targeted therapy in advanced non-small cell lung cancer: Current advances and future trends. Journal of Hematology. 2021;**14**(1):1-20

[21] Ramalingam SS, Vansteenkiste J, Planchard D, Cho BC, Gray JE, Ohe Y, et al. Overall survival with osimertinib in untreated, EGFR-mutated advanced NSCLC. The New England Journal of Medicine. 2020;**382**(1):41-50

[22] Lin JJ, Cardarella S, Lydon CA, Dahlberg SE, Jackman DM, Jänne PA, et al. Five-year survival in EGFR-mutant metastatic lung adenocarcinoma treated with EGFR-TKIs. Journal of Thoracic Oncology. 2016;**11**(4):556-565

[23] Musika W, Kamsa-Ard S, Jirapornkul C, Santong C, Phunmanee A. Lung cancer survival with current therapies and new targeted treatments: A Comprehensive Update from the Srinagarind Hospital-Based Cancer Registry from (2013 to 2017). Asian Pacific Journal of Cancer Prevention. 2021;**22**(8):2501-2507

[24] Garon EB, Hellmann MD, Rizvi NA, Carcereny E, Leighl NB, Ahn MJ, et al. Five-year overall survival for patients with advanced non–small-cell lung cancer treated with pembrolizumab: Results from the Phase I KEYNOTE-001 Study. Journal of Clinical Oncology. 2019;**37**(28):2518-2527

[25] Kantarjian H, Ravandi F, O'Brien S, Cortes J, Faderl S, Garcia-Manero G, et al. Intensive chemotherapy does not benefit most older patients (age 70 years or older) with acute myeloid leukemia. Blood. 2010;**116**(22):4422-4429

[26] Kumar SK, Rajkumar SV, Dispenzieri A, Lacy MQ, Hayman SR, Buadi FK, et al. Improved survival in multiple myeloma and the impact of novel therapies. Blood. 2008;**111**(5):2516-2520

[27] Yeh JC, Knight LS, Kane J, Doberman DJ, Gupta A, Smith TJ. Has there been a shift in use of subacute rehabilitation instead of hospice referral since immunotherapy has become

available? Journal of Oncology Practice/ American Society of Clinical Oncology. 2019;**15**(10):e849-e855

[28] Glisch C, Saeidzadeh S, Snyders T, Gilbertson-White S, Hagiwara Y, Lyckholm L. Immune checkpoint inhibitor use near the end of life: A Single-Center Retrospective Study. Journal of Palliative Medicine. Jul 2020;**23**(7):977-979

[29] Ghandourh WA. Palliative care in cancer: Managing patients' expectations. Journal of Medical Radiation Sciences. 2016;**63**(4):242-257

[30] Habib AR, Cronin AM, Earle CC, Tulsky JA, Mack JW, Abel GA, et al. How do blood cancer doctors discuss prognosis? Findings from a National Survey of Hematologic Oncologists. Journal of Palliative Medicine. Jun 2019;**22**(6):677-684

[31] Keating NL, Landrum MB, Rogers SO, Baum SK, Virnig BA, Huskamp HA, et al. Physician factors associated with discussions about end-of-life care. Cancer. 2010;**116**(4):998-1006

[32] Perez-Cruz PE, dos Santos R, Silva TB, Crovador CS, de Nascimento MS, Hall S, et al. Longitudinal temporal and probabilistic prediction of survival in a Cohort of patients with advanced cancer. Journal of Pain and Symptom Management. Nov 2014;**48**(5):875-882

[33] Cheon S, Agarwal A, Popovic M, Milakovic M, Lam M, Fu W, et al. The accuracy of clinicians' predictions of survival in advanced cancer: A review. Annals of Palliative Medicine. 2016;**5**(1):229-229

[34] Moss AH, Lunney JR, Culp S, Auber M, Kurian S, Rogers J, et al. Prognostic significance of the "Surprise" question in cancer patients. Journal of Palliative Medicine. 2010;**13**(7):837-840

[35] Maltoni M, Nanni O, Pirovano M, Scarpi E, Indelli M, Martini C, et al. Successful validation of the palliative prognostic score in terminally ill cancer patients. Journal of Pain and Symptom Management. 1999;**17**(4):240-247

[36] Pirovano M, Maltoni M, Nanni O, Marinari M, Indelli M, Zaninetta G, et al. A new palliative prognostic score: A first step for the staging of terminally ill cancer patients. Italian Multicenter and Study Group on Palliative Care. Journal of Pain and Symptom Management. 1999;**17**(4):231-239

[37] The Palliative Prognostic Score. Palliative Care Network of Wisconsin. 2022. Available from: https://www.mypcnow.org/fast-fact/the-palliative-prognostic-score/

[38] Glare PA, Eychmueller S, McMahon P. Diagnostic accuracy of the palliative prognostic score in hospitalized patients with advanced cancer. Journal of Clinical Oncology. 2004;**22**(23):4823-4828

[39] Yoon SJ, Suh SY, Hui D, Choi SE, Tatara R, Watanabe H, et al. Accuracy of the palliative prognostic score with or without clinicians' prediction of survival in patients with far advanced cancer. Journal of Pain and Symptom Management. 2021;**61**(6):1180-1187

[40] Anderson F, Downing GM, Hill J, Casorso L, Lerch N. Palliative performance scale (PPS): A new tool. Journal of Palliative Care. 1996;**12**(1):5-11

[41] Wilner LS, Arnold RM. The palliative performance scale #125. Journal of Palliative Medicine. 2006;**9**(4):994-994

[42] Downing GM. Q&A Manual, Instructions & Definitions for Use of Palliative Performance Scale (PPSv2). July 24, 2020

[43] Lau F, Downing GM, Lesperance M, Shaw J, Kuziemsky C. Use of palliative performance scale in end-of-life prognostication. Journal of Palliative Medicine. 2006;**9**(5):1066-1075

[44] Morita T, Tsunoda J, Inoue S, Chihara S. Validity of the palliative performance scale from a survival perspective. Journal of Pain and Symptom Management. 1999;**18**(1):2-3

[45] Morita T, Tsunoda J, Inoue S, Chihara S. The Palliative Prognostic Index: A scoring system for survival prediction of terminally ill cancer patients. Support Care Cancer. 1999;7(3):128-133

[46] Stone PC, Lund S. Predicting prognosis in patients with advanced cancer. Annals of Oncology. 2007;**18**(6):971-976

[47] Stone CA, Tiernan E, Dooley BA. Prospective validation of the palliative prognostic index in patients with cancer. Journal of Pain and Symptom Management. 2008;**35**(6):617-622

[48] Yun YH, Heo DS, Heo BY, Yoo TW, Bae JM, Ahn SH. Development of terminal cancer prognostic score as an index in terminally ill cancer patients. Oncology Reports. 2001;**8**(4):795-800

[49] Bruera E, Miller MJ, Kuehn N, MacEachern T, Hanson J. Estimate of survival of patients admitted to a palliative care unit: A prospective study. Journal of Pain and Symptom Management. 1992;7(2):82-86

[50] Charlson ME, Pompei P, Ales KL, MacKenzie CR. A new method of classifying prognostic comorbidity in longitudinal studies: Development and validation. Journal of Chronic Diseases. 1987;**40**(5):373-383

[51] Asano T, Yamada S, Fujii T, Yabusaki N, Nakayama G, Sugimoto H, et al. The Charlson age comorbidity index predicts prognosis in patients with resected pancreatic cancer. International Journal of Surgery. 2017;**39**:169-175

[52] Chien SH, Yao M, Li CC, Chang PY, Yu MS, Huang CE, et al. Charlson comorbidity index predicts outcomes of elderly after allogeneic hematopoietic stem cell transplantation for acute myeloid leukemia and myelodysplastic syndrome. Journal of Formosan Medical Association. 2021;**120**(12):2144-2152

[53] Singh B, Bhaya M, Stern J, Roland JT, Zimbler M, Rosenfeld RM, et al. Validation of the Charlson comorbidity index in patients with head and neck cancer: A multi-institutional study. The Laryngoscope. 1997;**107** (11 Pt 1):1469-1475

[54] Zhao L, Leung LH, Wang J, Li H, Che J, Liu L, et al. Association between Charlson comorbidity index score and outcome in patients with stage IIIB-IV non-small cell lung cancer. BMC Pulmonary Medicine. 2017;**17**(1):112

[55] Maltoni M, Caraceni A, Brunelli C, Broeckaert B, Christakis N, Eychmueller S, et al. Prognostic factors in advanced cancer patients: Evidence-based clinical recommendations--a study by the Steering Committee of the European Association for Palliative Care. Journal of Clinical Oncology: Official Journal of the American Society of Clinical Oncology. 2005;**23**(25):6240-6248

[56] Chu C, Anderson R, White N, Stone P. Prognosticating for adult patients with advanced incurable cancer: A needed oncologist skill. Current Treatment Options in Oncology. 2020;**21**(1):5

[57] Button E, Cardona M, Huntley K, Gavin NC, LeBlanc TW, Olsen A, et al. Clinicians' understanding of preferences and values of people with hematological malignancies at the end of life: Concurrent surveys. Journal of Palliative Medicine. Apr 19, 2022. DOI: 10.1089/jpm.2021.0490. PMID: 35443803 [Epub ahead of print]

[58] Hagerty RG, Butow PN, Ellis PA, Lobb EA, Pendlebury S, Leighl N, et al. Cancer patient preferences for communication of prognosis in the metastatic setting. Journal of Clinical Oncology: Official Journal of the American Society of Clinical Oncology. 2004;**22**(9):1721-1730

[59] Parker SM, Clayton JM, Hancock K, Walder S, Butow PN, Carrick S, et al. A systematic review of prognostic/end-of-life communication with adults in the advanced stages of a life-limiting illness: Patient/caregiver preferences for the content, style, and timing of information. Journal of Pain and Symptom Management. 2007;**34**(1):81-93

[60] van der Velden NCA, Meijers MC, Han PKJ, van Laarhoven HWM, Smets EMA, Henselmans I. The effect of prognostic communication on patient outcomes in palliative cancer care: A systematic review. Current Treatment Options in Oncology. 2020;**21**(5):40

[61] Westendorp J, Evers AWM, Stouthard JML, Budding J, van der Wall E, Plum NMF, et al. Mind your words: Oncologists' communication that potentially harms patients with advanced cancer: A survey on patient perspectives. Cancer. 2022;**128**(5):1133-1140

[62] Medendorp NM, Stiggelbout AM, Aalfs CM, Han PKJ, Smets EMA, Hillen MA. A scoping review of practice recommendations for clinicians' communication of uncertainty. Health Expectations: International Journal of Public Participation in Health Care Health Policy. 2021;**24**(4):1025-1043

[63] Mori M, Fujimori M, Ishiki H, Nishi T, Hamano J, Otani H, et al. Adding a wider range and "Hope for the Best, and Prepare for the Worst" statement: Preferences of patients with cancer for prognostic communication. The Oncologist. 2019;**24**(9):e943-e952

[64] Kruser JM, Nabozny MJ, Steffens NM, Brasel KJ, Campbell TC, Gaines ME, et al. "Best Case/Worst Case": Qualitative evaluation of a novel communication tool for difficult in-the-moment surgical decisions. Journal of the American Geriatrics Society. 2015;**63**(9):1805-1811

[65] Taylor LJ, Nabozny MJ, Steffens NM, Tucholka JL, Brasel KJ, Johnson SK, et al. A framework to improve surgeon communication in high-stakes surgical decisions: Best case/worst case. JAMA Surgery. 2017;**152**(6):531-538

[66] LeBlanc TW, Temel JS, Helft PR. "How Much Time Do I Have?": Communicating prognosis in the era of exceptional responders. American Society of Clinical Oncology. 2018;**38**:787-794

[67] Childers JW, Back AL, Tulsky JA, Arnold RM. REMAP: A framework for goals of care conversations. Journal of Oncology Practice/ American Society of Clinical Oncology. 2017;**13**(10):e844-e850

[68] Lakin JR, Tulsky JA, Bernacki RE. Time out before talking: Communication as a medical procedure. Annals of Internal Medicine. 2021;**174**(1):96-97